ESCAPING THE PAIN MATRIX

THE FUTURE OF PAIN RELIEF

DR. DANIEL R. WOODRUFF, D.C

Foreword

My wife, Marty, and I have our permanent home on the Old West Side of Ann Arbor, Michigan. We also have a home in Lewiston, Michigan, 400 miles round trip, which we travel to and from frequently during the year. We heard from an old friend of ours, who was a patient of Dr. Woodruff, that he might be a fit for me and my lower back issues. Marty and I set up an appointment with Dr. Woodruff at his Lewiston location to see if he could help me.

In the past, I have had many surgeries due to playing contact sports from the mid-1960s to the 1980s.

- Football, in both games and training, for the Detroit Public School Football League 1967-1969 at Cooley High School. My senior year, I was co-captain and most valuable player as a linebacker.
- Schoolcraft Junior College 1970-72: 1972 State champion in Handball.
- United States Marine Corps Officers Candidate School 1974; in 1976 as a 1st Lieutenant based out of the 2nd Marine Division, Camp Lejeune, North Carolina, I played rugby around the world.
- Graduate student at the University of Michigan in the 1980s. Rugby National Finals 1982: I was an All-American, and U of M was the national runner-up for universities in North America.

Surgeries happened during the time from the late 1960s to 2017. They were all conducted in Ann Arbor.

- Left knee ligament
- Right knee replacement
- Left and right hip replacements
- Left and right shoulder replacements
- Spinal fusion C3-C6
- Left wrist fusion

My injuries dramatically affected my life. I know many others have dealt with similar injuries. Although surgeries helped me, as time went on, my medical issues affected my mobility, posture, and pain levels. Due to quality-of-life concerns, I decided to look at a different alternative with Dr. Woodruff—Neuromuscular Modulation (Vibrate-A-Way's more scientific name for the vibrational technique).

While at my first appointment with Dr. Woodruff, we learned about the relationship between the brain and injury (pain). It made complete sense to us! I had a new goal: setting up a home program using Neuromuscular Modulation (the Vibrate-A-Way ™ program), which should help me have better posture and balance again.

With training, Marty thought she could help me at home. We started with 3 to 4 training sessions with Dr. Woodruff and read his written information. Marty showed Dr. Woodruff what she learned, and he approved for us to begin the process of working at home. We began home sessions 5-6 times per week. I checked in with Dr. Woodruff face-to-face every 3 months. In addition, I was able to have contact via email if I had any questions or concerns. We were all very excited about this opportunity—a great chance to get better.

Marty was well-trained by Dr. Woodruff. Although I continue treatment at the Michigan Pain Clinic, participating in the Vibrate-A-Way™ program at home has helped me more than my treatment at the pain clinic alone. The combination of medical modalities has helped me improve in 2022. I am very happy with both applications. Adding Dr. Woodruff's at-home plan has been a marvelous addition in support of my pain issues. We are looking forward to continued improvement and learning more from Dr. Woodruff's published work.

Ian
Davis Chapman 2022

"You take the blue pill—the story ends, you wake up in your bed and believe whatever you want to believe. You take the red pill—you stay in Wonderland, and I show you how deep the rabbit hole goes. Remember, all I'm offering is the truth. Nothing more."

-- Morpheus, *The Matrix*

Introduction

*"What is **real**? How do you define '**real**'? If you're talking about what you can feel, what you can smell, taste and see, then '**real**' is simply electrical signals interpreted by your brain. However, you have to understand, most people are not ready to be unplugged."*

-- Morpheus, *The Matrix*

So much of our life is shaped by popular culture. Not only does it shape what we buy, but also how we think and how we see the world around us. Of course, we notice this with controversial issues that are currently in our headlines. The reach and impact of popular culture shapes our values and belief systems. Those who wish to promote their belief systems commonly utilize the media—both traditional and social—to spread their ideology. It is only too easy to understand that if one can tap into its power, one can change the world merely by changing popular culture. There are many definitions of the word *culture*. The one I like and will share with you is as follows: culture is a way of life of a group of people—the behaviors, beliefs, values, and symbols that they accept, generally without thinking about them, and that are passed along by communication and imitation from one generation to the next.

A cultural "norm" is a belief, value or behavior that society accepts as correct and normal. Cultural norms allow us to function in society in an orderly manner. Values such as kindness and generosity are deemed good and acceptable. On the other hand, others, such as greed and jealousy, are viewed in a negative light.

However, while these behaviors may be seen as good or bad; it doesn't necessarily mean that they are normal or abnormal. For example, taxes: some view that system as bad and others see it as good; yet, both can typically agree that taxes are normal and necessary for government and society to run. Of course, the room for argument is how much tax is needed, where the funds are to be spent, and who benefits. But, alas, that is a subject for another book by another author.

Cultural norms can be a hindrance, a reliable guide, or they can even be both. How do we know which it is for any given belief, value or behavior? That is a conundrum. Can a cultural norm or belief that has endured decades of acceptance be wrong? Obviously, the answer to that is yes: you just have to look at the horrible history of the institutions of racism or sexism as a blatant example, but that is picking low-lying fruit. There are many more examples that are forgotten and less extreme.

Since this book is about health and healthcare, let's use an example of that. Prevalent in the 1940s through the early 1970s, cigarette smoking not only was accepted but promoted. Famous athletes, actors and even doctors extolled the benefits of smoking. As a result, cigarette smoking was viewed as a habit, not a destructive addiction. Only when research proved the detrimental impact to health from smoking did the attitudes and social mores change. The tobacco industry fought long and hard to downplay and challenge the validity of these findings. When this approach failed, they then made it about an individual's right to choose to smoke. This approach allowed the cigarette industry to survive; however, after much litigation from individuals and the government, the tobacco giants financially settled and provided warnings and public service announcements about the dangers of smoking.

Just because an institution has been in existence for a long time does not necessarily mean that it is correct or beneficial. "Pop" culture has the ability to sustain or tear down any long-established institution, whether it be a physical one or an emotional or intellectual one. In fact, one can take "pop" culture to not only mean "popular" culture but also "populous" culture. Not only are we influenced by the traditional instruments of cultural change like the internet, social media and television, but we are also influenced by our peers who have been influenced. So, when I think of pop culture I think of these two aspects.

For these reasons, it is difficult for many to see that the information they have about a subject is slanted towards something or somebody who has a vested interest. Would you expect a research study conducted about the health benefits of oranges to be negative if it was funded by an orange growers' association? Of course not. This occurs with more studies than you may care to believe. It takes money to conduct research: you must pay for the team of scientists and equipment vital to the study. Well, where does this money come from? If I were a wealthy billionaire, would I just out-of-the-blue decide to fund research about oranges? What do you think? Many, if not most times, this research is conducted by an organization who wishes to promote the efficacy and validity of their product or idea. The problem is that if you try to chase the funding, it goes through so many faux "think tanks," foundations and other "scientific" organizations, it will be very hard to pinpoint who's really funding the study.

The media—traditional or social—will label this automatically as a scientific study that proves oranges are good for health. Most of us—myself excluded, because I am in the minority—will accept this at face value. I mean, come on, how can you argue that oranges aren't good for you? But have you read the research conducted making that claim? Have you read other research, some of which may state that oranges are bad for you? Most of us don't. Most of us don't have time to. I get it. However, it is our blind acceptance of the word "science" put before any idea that may give us a wrong belief or false information. When you combine that with the internet and television promotion of this science, all of a sudden you have a pop culture belief taking form.

Yet, it is hard to *unplug* from the influence of what pop culture labels as correct/incorrect, good/bad, and right/wrong. Most times, what we are exposed to is only one side of an issue. In today's society, we no longer have tolerance of other viewpoints. Oppositional ideas or theories are violently attacked and discredited as ridiculous or morally wrong. The popular pressure to embrace a viewpoint has become heightened.

Thus, to *unplug* from a belief or "fact" that doesn't seem right, is hard to do. There is far less support and information on opposing ideas. Not only is there a paucity of support for an alternative view, but many times there is vehement support *for* the popular view. It is, in fact, very difficult to search for what is **"real"** when what is accepted is so strongly and emotionally defended.

I have always been a big fan of dichotomy and irony. I find it to be the head-scratch of life. It is for this reason that I titled my book, *The Pain Matrix*. Not only do I wish to draw upon the Pop Culture influence of the movie *The Matrix,* but I want to use it to expose the influence of Pop Culture in musculoskeletal healthcare.

In the movie, people lived what they thought were normal lives. In reality, they were contained in pods, being used as electrical energy to supply the computers who, through artificial intelligence, gained control over the humans. The main character, Neo, lived his life like the others, yet he felt like something wasn't quite right. It was this desire to find out the truth that led him to Morpheus. Morpheus showed Neo that his existence was provided for him in the Matrix. The Matrix was, in fact, a false reality. It was not a real life but an appeasement to the senses. It provided the stimulus to them so that the humans thought they were living. At first, Neo didn't want to believe it, nor could he; but he eventually acknowledged that what he was told was living, was not.

In this book, I hope to show you how the healthcare system has been, in a way, a matrix to us. They have appeased our senses with temporary pain relief or false solutions, while not addressing the true problem. Yet, there is a way! The answers are out there. Unfortunately, these answers have been fragmented and dispersed throughout thousands of pages of research. I have spent the better part of my life searching, gathering and synthesizing this data. I have spent years researching and experimenting to find long-lasting solutions to musculoskeletal problems.

Throughout this process, I made one amazing discovery: it is so simple, you will doubt that it could work, but it does! The answer lies not in our future but from our past. The answer lies not in technology but in the simple basic sciences. In fact, the answer is so simple, that no matter your background or experience, you can have and use this discovery!

"The answer is out there, Neo, and it's looking for you, and it will find you if you want it to."

-- Trinity, *The Matrix*

XIV

Notice

The techniques and protocols of Vibrate-A-Way, Inc. or its program are not medical applications. They are not intended to cure, treat, mitigate, diagnose or prevent disease, and they have not been reviewed by the FDA. The information on these pages is for reference and educational purposes only. It should not be treated as a substitute for professional medical advice, diagnosis or treatment. You should always seek such advice from a qualified medical professional.

Chapter 1:
You & the Pain Matrix

We've been brainwashed. You see, we follow the same pattern over and over. It all starts when we feel pain or dysfunction in a joint or a muscle, somewhere on the body, and our first response is, "Maybe it will go away." We all do that. We try to wait it out. Some people will wait 3 days, some people 3 weeks, and some people 3 months. When we have come to the conclusion that it will not go away on its own, most of the population will then go to their medical doctor. The course of treatment for an injury is generally the same: first, there will be a brief examination and maybe an x-ray on a joint that is affected. We will then be prescribed steroids, muscle relaxants or maybe pain medication (although the medical community is shying away from narcotics and honestly rightfully so). We will be told to come back if the pain or dysfunction doesn't go away. Finally, when the pain is still there after two weeks have passed, and the prescription has run out, we go back.

Since there is no improvement, we are going to be sent to physical therapy. You see, most insurance companies, in order to pay for an MRI, require that the patient receives physical therapy first. "Cost containment" is the vital phrase that they use. We might go to physical therapy anywhere from 4 to 8 weeks, 2 to 3 times a week, and it helps: we can move better, and the pain is diminishing. But the course of treatment ends--whether the insurance runs out or the treatment has reached "maximum medical improvement." We are given a packet of home exercises and told to just keep doing these exercises because they will either maintain or even improve our condition. But, let's be real with each other, as we are in this book and as we always will be: we don't do them. If I were to give an educated guess, I would say 95% of the people that are given home exercises don't do them. I know I don't. You see, generally, there are unrealistic expectations placed on us by the provider to do 12 different home exercises twice a day. I don't have an hour-and-a-half of my time to go through these exercises, and so what happens is that we might start off fairly consistently, dwindle down, and then we just don't do them at all.

Next, we go back to the medical provider and say, "It didn't work. It still hurts." Now, they can order the MRI. So, when we get to that stage we are looking at one of two solution paths. The first option, pain management (which is a dirty phrase for anybody who currently is going through pain management, and we will get into that later in the book), or the other option, surgery. At this point, some people decide, "Uh-oh! Well, I have to try everything before I let them cut me open!" And it's generally at that exact point when they will go see a chiropractor or another alternative therapist.

With chiropractic, it's essentially the same pattern. Chiropractors will adjust people 2 to 3 times a week, for 4 to 8 weeks, and it works. The pain or dysfunction improves, but after about 2 weeks, it comes back. You see, that's the very reason why I almost quit chiropractic. I would work on people, improve them, but you know what? Every 2 weeks to a month, they would come back with the same problems. I'm a person who believes that every story has a beginning, a middle, and an end; *and my healthcare should also have a beginning, a middle, and an end.* To continually go on dealing with pain was not a suitable answer to me—not as a patient or as a provider. I was frustrated with the limitations that my occupation as a chiropractor provided, and it was that frustration which motivated me to create Vibrate-A-Way™.

Vibrate-A-Way™ is *the future's solution to an age-old problem of musculoskeletal pain and dysfunction.* As you may already be realizing, we have followed the same model or system of assessment and treatment for musculoskeletal care for several decades. I call this entire system *the Pain Matrix*. The following definitions are from the Oxford Languages Dictionary:

Pain: physical suffering or discomfort caused by illness or injury

Matrix: an environment or material in which something develops

Standard musculoskeletal healthcare is a part of this Matrix, as they are supposed to have the knowledge and technology to treat musculoskeletal pain and dysfunction. You're inside of the Pain Matrix, too, because you automatically follow the same patterns as you've been taught (or programmed) to follow, by the standard healthcare component of the Pain Matrix. Yet, how effective have these patterns been to treat dysfunction and relieve pain? Albert Einstein is credited with this phrase that is so appropriate here: "The definition of insanity is doing something the same way over and over again and expecting a different result." And that is what musculoskeletal care has been: we might try to advance our approach by utilizing technology to improve our assessment, but it is the same in the end. You understand, to fix a problem in a different way, you first must *see* the problem in a different way. If you can recognize the existence of the Pain Matrix, then this is your first step in freeing yourself from its grasp. Let's look together at the problem of dysfunction and pain and examine it through a new lens.

In this book, as you go forth, I am going to make a big ask of you: you must drop any preconceived notions of musculoskeletal pain. All that you knew was "right"; what your friends or your healthcare providers tell you; whatever they might know or claim to know, is the opinion of the standard healthcare system within the Pain Matrix. Paradigms are constantly shifting and changing. After all, there was a time when scientists believed the earth was flat. There were fears that when the sun went over the horizon, it had disappeared completely, and rituals would be performed so that the sun would come up again the next day. Well, we became enlightened, and we realized the earth is round and the *sun* actually revolves around the *earth*. A new way of thinking that explains things. Relax! The sun will come back out. But *then* a smart man named Galileo said, "No, you know what? The *earth* actually revolves around the *sun*." That got Galileo Galilei in trouble with the holy Roman church because, you see, by saying the earth revolved around the sun, it diminished God because He created earth, which means everything should revolve around the earth. So, Galileo changed the paradigm of how we looked at things. It landed him in house arrest for the rest of his life; but with his research, his gazing into the stars and making observations, he was able to see that the earth did revolve around the sun, as did the other planets. But, because the previously-held Matrix of his time saw that the earth was the center point and everything else revolved around it, they did not want to hear the new information. And, many times, we are that way.

> *"I can only show you the door. You're the one that has to walk through it."* – Morpheus, *the Matrix*

If light is shed on the deficiencies of the status quo, why do so many resist following the truth and making the change? Why do we feel a tendency to defy progression? We hear stories, and although the account was not witnessed firsthand, we have a tendency to accept it verbatim, without question. Although we have never done any research, we trust it. But what is the source of that information? What is the validity of that information? Was that information slanted toward one view or another?

I have to share my version one of my favorite stories, here. I have to say it's a story because this is actually another example of "fact or fiction" controversy. Either way, it makes you think. The story tells of scientists who wanted to determine the effects of negative reinforcement on monkeys, so they placed five monkeys in a room. In the center of the room were blocks to climb upon. A banana would lower down from the ceiling, and the first time a monkey went up on the blocks to get that banana, he and the others were sprayed with cold water for a length of time. They made a few more attempts, and every time, the monkeys would get sprayed with water. By then, any time a monkey would get an idea that maybe he would try it, the other monkeys would basically knock him off the blocks and kind of beat on him. So, what the researchers then did was to take out one of the original six monkeys and replace it with a new monkey. Seeing the banana being lowered, this new monkey tried to climb up, but the other monkeys beat him up. No water was sprayed. The monkeys just beat him up before he could get the banana. And so, one by one, they replaced the original monkeys to the point that none of the five monkeys that remained in the room had never been sprayed with water when they grabbed the banana. Anytime a new monkey was introduced into the group and tried to reach the banana, the other monkeys would beat him up, <u>even though they never had the negative reinforcement of the water.</u> You know, if monkeys could talk and we could have asked them, "Why are you beating up that monkey?" I bet their answer would be, "Well, because that's how it's always been done around here." And I believe that is the answer to why our Pain Matrix is allowed to exist. **That's how it's always been done.** You understand, anything in this world that we accept as tradition or the "correct way" always started as a new idea. It was initially met with skepticism, but it became accepted as people were willing to try it—to embrace it.

I feel that there are two kinds of people in this world: the ones who want to be proven right and the ones who want to be proven wrong. You can read this book and say, "Yeah, I don't think this is going to work." Or you can be one of those that says, "This is the answer I have been waiting for!" And to you I say (one of my favorite phrases), "Whether you think you can or can't, you are absolutely right!" Whether you think this will or won't work for you or your loved ones, you are absolutely right. So, as you continue on into this book, I want you to open your mind to release any limiting, preconceived systems of thinking, regarding what should be done for your pain and your dysfunction, and be willing to embrace something new. If it weren't for new concepts and ideas, the word "innovation" wouldn't be around. The world is full of innovations. We see them almost every day. Healthcare has been doing the same thing the same way for far too long when it comes to musculoskeletal care, and so have we. It's time for fresh, new innovation and new ways of looking at musculoskeletal problems. New ways of combating them. And this is what Vibrate-A-Way™ can do.

Chapter 2:
The Notion of Singles

In the first chapter, I briefly hit upon the normal route that we go through with our standard and even some alternative healthcare when it comes to musculoskeletal conditions. Quite simply, our healthcare system, inside the Pain Matrix, is really set up and based upon this notion: for every problem, there is a single cause with a single effect; therefore, we have a single solution. The reason for your pain is "this," and here is a medication. The reason for your problem is "this," so do these exercises/stretches. The reason for your problem is "this"; I am going to adjust you. Whichever discipline it may be, it tends to follow the same pattern, and that is *single cause, single effect, and single solution.*

Another thing with old Pain Matrix logic is something I call "blaming an old culprit." I believe it was in the movie *Casablanca* where they told them to round up the "usual suspects," and that is kind of how we treat what we're feeling when it comes to musculoskeletal problems. We always want to blame an old culprit—the usual suspect. There are people who had a disc herniation or bulge from 20 or 25 years ago, and—to hear them talk—that injury still causes problems. Then, for another, there is an old high school football injury on an elbow or a shoulder or whatever it might be. We like to blame the old culprits, so anytime we feel pain in an area, we bring them back up. Here they come! Round up the usual suspects. It's the old football injury. And we are made to believe that.

We have been taught to think in terms of identifying the single cause, so we can tie it in to the single effect, so we can have our single solution. To give you a better example, if you have a sore shoulder, the first question is, "Did you do anything to it?" or "What did you do?" Now, I am not faulting the healthcare practitioner. You have to know if something or an injury did take place: is there acute trauma or is it chronic pain? But, often, the very first question is, "Did you do anything?" Consequently, our brain learns the pattern of directly finding the single cause. Something that drives me crazy in practice is when a patient wants to know what they could have done to cause their condition. And they will keep searching for the answer. They will keep searching. They will keep questioning, "What could I have done?" thinking about this, that, and the other. Anybody who is close to me knows that I have a go-to answer to that: "It doesn't matter how the zebra got in the bathtub, we need to get the zebra out of the bathtub. It's not my job to figure out how he got there; it is my job to get him out of there." And when I tell them that, most people will say to me, "Well, if I knew what I did, I could prevent it from happening again." Of course, I have to respond, "You know that when you lift heavy objects, you should always bend with your knees and not lift with your back. Do you do that every time?" After they admit they don't, I ask rhetorically: "You know the speed limit on the highway is 55 mph. Do you travel 55 every time?" Well, I'm pretty sure that answer is no, too. As you can see, we are stuck in that Matrix's archaic method of thought of "let's find the cause, so we can find the effect, and then I can give you a single solution." I mean, after all, the insurance industry is built upon giving a proper diagnosis. Before you can do anything, you have to have a diagnosis. You have to tell them what is causing the problem. I understand you have to know what it is you are treating, in a way, but the single cause has become more of the focus.

Another focus is on pain, itself, and people's perception of pain. We'll get into pain versus dysfunction/function, later; but our need to get out of pain—to finally get relief—is a major perpetuator of the Pain Matrix. After all, without pain, there is no Pain Matrix!

Back to the focus on having to find a diagnosis, the Pain Matrix has created an over-reliance on technology. Granted, we have advanced our technology—the technology that we have to see inside the body and to gather data is incredible. But how we utilize the information from that technology hasn't changed: we're still seeing it and analyzing it through the lens of finding that single cause, and let's take the leap of it causing that one, single effect. It's dangerous to put all of our eggs into that basket, much less all of our health and well-being.

We choose our healthcare solution, in many ways, like we choose a religious denomination. It's almost a belief system. Well-meaning people frequently tell me they "believe" in chiropractic. Well, it's not a belief system. It's been around for over 120 years, and trust me, if it wasn't effective or legitimate, the US government would have shut it down a long time ago. On the flip side, I will have patients in my clinic who criticize medical doctors for prescribing "poison," saying they are nothing but drug-pushers; and that's wrong, too. You see, there is an appropriateness to all of our treatments. If I needed to pound a nail into a piece of wood, I would not grab a screwdriver.

Conversely, if I needed to screw something in, I wouldn't grab a hammer. Logical, right? However, we sometimes use different criteria when choosing our healthcare solution. We may go off of belief in certain fields or methods or base our decision on past experiences (even the past experiences of family and friends), and that can be dangerous. Decisions based on emotion and not logic when it comes to these matters can lead to trouble—it can lead to the wrong decision being made. Therefore, I always remind any patient to make their decision based on what they know is best for themselves, and that is based on concrete information that they have gathered.

Speaking of gathering information, let's talk about information-gathering in the world of the internet. Information and the gathering of information is a good thing. After all, if I didn't have access to the information I did via the Internet, I could have never, ever come up with Vibrate-A-Way™. But just like anything else in this world, too much information can be harmful, and which information can be trusted as truth? I often joke with my friends and colleagues that I am amazed by how many "doctors" come through my door in a day. Between WebMD and Dr. Google, the diagnoses that patients come up with when they come to see me are incredible! It seems to be a trend because they follow this pattern (another pattern!): first, they will generally take the first few diagnoses that come up in their search that relate to their symptoms and assume it must be one of those. From there, they narrow it down to the one diagnosis that's the harshest. A great example of this is a person who comes in with shoulder pain they've been suffering with for three months. They know they need surgery because it is definitely a torn rotator cuff. They have their single cause, they have their single effect, and their single solution, as they were programmed to find.

Unfortunately, it is the worst-case scenario for that shoulder, and that is because we have all been indoctrinated into the thinking of the Pain Matrix. How sad, right? What if the information that person gathered included a scientific study that was essentially "research in a vacuum," isolated from pertinent facts, and which only purpose was to prove or disprove a single cause/effect or solution? The information obviously wouldn't have taken into consideration this person's situation; but because this person feels shoulder pain, and the study was about shoulder pain and had concluded that the rotator cuff was torn, they made a wrong assumption that this "science" applies to their situation, even though they're not inside that vacuum with the research study.

Moving forward, I want to open your eyes to the scientific truth of a new way of seeing and thinking--not only about the problem, but about how we can utilize those truths for our *solutions*. We first must awaken to the reality of the Pain Matrix, itself. Next, given this new knowledge, we have to decide whether to stay and "live with it" or to *escape* and be free to live our best lives we'd only dreamed about before we were awakened. Which pill will you choose?

Chapter 3:

Channeling Your Inner Galileo

(A New Lens)

I hope I have exposed to you how musculoskeletal care is performed within the Pain Matrix: its method of *viewing* the problem, which leads to old approaches of trying to *solve* the problem and that it is all *ineffective*. Now, any fool can point out trouble as the event is going bad. That is easy. But the real art—the really hard part—is to come up with a remedy to the situation. It sorts out the wheat from the chaff, if you will. In this chapter, I want to start by presenting to you that new lens to look through, a new way of viewing the same old problems. First off, we have to break the "single cause, the single effect, and the single solution" approach. This approach lies at the heart of most of our problems, as I've mentioned—a lot, I know. To explain, we are big into cause-and-effect so that the situation makes logical sense to our brain. What drives us crazy is if our shoulder hurts, and we do not think we did anything to it. Then we're befuddled. The human body (especially the brain) is too complex for such a simple approach. *Our brain is a master computer: it handles everything. We know that it is in charge of all of our bodily functions, our organ systems; but when it comes to the musculoskeletal system, we choose not to enter the brain into the equation.* If we see a doctor for a knee problem that's been bothering us for a few months or so, the first thing that every health care provider is going to do is to look at the knee, itself.

And we tie in some kind of recent trauma that we think could be the cause of it. If we can't find recent trauma, we start digging for old trauma. If tests or scans are ordered, they're focused only on the knee. All Pain Matrix.

Allow me to present to you: "the brain." The brain is an integral part of this equation and controls the body more than we ever knew: it is continually changing our posture and our movement, based on stimuli it perceives from the outside world and the internal environment of our body. We are all given a posture as human beings: we are bipedal animals—upright. Posture is more than just cosmetics. Many people look at a picture and notice their posture; they may say something like, "Oh, I look horrible! I'm all stooped over, and my head is always leaning to the left when I take a picture!" Well, there is more to it than simply how you appear. To expound, *posture is the beginning and end point of all motion*. If you have proper posture, you will have proper motion. Proper posture means an absence of dysfunction and an absence of pain. After all, if your joints are lined up correctly and moving properly, they will not create friction. Improper *posture* means improper *movement*. Improper movement leads to friction, degeneration, pain and eventual surgeries.

The brain controls our movement and our posture, based on outlying stimuli—whether from outside or inside; therefore, to protect a perceived area of problem or to make us more stable, the brain will change our posture. For example, if I have a painful right knee that I'm having a hard time bending, I will walk differently: I will have a limp, or I will bear more weight on the opposite leg, in order to protect that knee. The other factor that you have to take into consideration with the changes in posture is that the change in posture, in the bigger picture, is *changing our physics*. Whether you like to admit it or not, our bodies are nothing more than machines. We are eleven organ systems and a soul. Our internal organs are protected by a rigid, bony structure that is surrounded by muscles for movement and flesh to encase it all. That's the cold hard facts of it, but, nevertheless, we are a machine. We are not made of steel, but we are made of carbon. The laws of physics, which are universal and apply to all things, apply also to us; yet, in the old approaches of the Pain Matrix, we didn't think about the physics of the body. We only thought about the symptoms of the affected area, of the joint—whatever it might have been. You have to realize, we've been trained not to look at or treat the body and brain as one continuous unit: we isolate and separate. I can't tell you how many times I have been able to take away someone's knee pain in my clinic by working on their shoulders! Now, that might not make sense to you, but it makes perfect sense to me for the reason that everything is tied in together. You know the old saying, "everything is connected," but we really can't appreciate just how connected everything is. Everything *is* connected! Therefore, if you have an improperly functioning shoulder, it will affect a knee, an ankle. So, let's figure out why it's all so connected, shall we?

In God's great design of the human body, we were basically equipped or programmed with override systems. For instance, if I broke an ankle, I would still be able to ambulate somehow—a survival mechanism, if you will. We all have failsafe overrides in case of problems. *When the body is injured, the brain will accommodate to protect that injury*, except the brain doesn't make an accommodation just around the area of injury, alone: the brain will also change the rest of the body. It diffuses it throughout the whole body so nothing is too sudden, nothing is too drastic. It's going to do 10% in one area, 5% in another, 10% in still another area, and so on, limiting the motion by those percentages. It will change our posture. In such manner does the brain, *throughout the whole body.*

Alright, so we recognize that the brain is continually changing our posture and our movement, not only to protect areas of injury, but to also ensure that we can still move, while remaining stable in our stance and in our movement. Come again? The brain is not only going to accommodate to protect an injury, but it is also going to accommodate to provide an "override" way of moving, while providing stability to our altered posture and movement. Let's talk about physics and how we have to abide by the laws of physics. *This—the physics—is what gets affected when the brain makes accommodations.* For example, center of gravity. Center of gravity, as we know, is the center load that weighs down on us. Now, in the human body, and from a sideways perspective, it goes downward through our ear, shoulder, hip, knee and our anklebone. However, if—due to an injury—we are forward of that, then our center of gravity is off. Weight-bearing is disproportionate to how it should be. It looks like this: if you are bent or tilted forward up high so that your head and shoulders are forward of your ankles, you will be improperly bearing more weight on your knees, resulting in knee pain. If your pelvis is higher on one side as opposed to the other, then you'll bear more weight on the lower side; consequently, more friction is created in the weight-bearing leg. Then, because of this, the joint system that is used when you ambulate, or walk, can't do it the way it should. As a result of the joint system malfunction, instead of the leg swinging freely like a pendulum, it will go into more of a rotational stride. We'll talk more about that, later; but did you notice more than one effect? Does the cause of the accommodation really matter? Or do we simply need a solution to our machine's physics problem, so it can function properly and painlessly again?

These concepts change how we identify the reason we feel the pain in our body. What happens is this: when the brain makes accommodations to repetitive use/motion, injuries or trauma, it's going to do it in such a manner that the brain will tighten up some muscles and shut down other muscles. It will make some muscles work harder because—if a joint can't move well, and the brain has to protect it—the brain will further limit the motion of that joint. Creating motion in a joint is work, and work is a form of energy. Einstein told us that energy cannot be destroyed: it can only be changed, moved, or altered; therefore, the work that an area of the body used to do—but now doesn't—has to be transferred somewhere else.

This physics lesson leads us to another paradigm shift, and it's this—ready? This is a big one. *Many times, in an area of chronic pain or chronic dysfunction, the problem isn't the side that is symptomatic: it is the side that is not symptomatic.* This is another concept worth repeating: again, the side that is symptomatic, showing pain or dysfunction of movement, in most cases, is not the side that is the problem! It is the opposite side. Why? Because the opposite side is not working. The side that is painful is working too hard. It has to pick up the extra work energy of the side that isn't moving properly. You ask, why, if an area is not working, would it be dysfunctional? Why would it cause pain? It's not moving. There are no chances for it to create inflammation, abnormal movement or joint dysfunction. It's simply not moving. Your answer is that the other side—or the opposite joint, however you want to look at it—has to pick up the work. And that creates more pain. Not only does this apply to the left and right sides of the body but also the top to bottom. That is why I have said that I am able to fix a knee by working on a shoulder. It is because of the transference of work that has been limited by the knee. Therefore, the assumption we have to get away from is that the area of pain is the area of problem. Most cases it's not, and that is why I feel the biggest error in viewing the problem inside the Pain Matrix is that the area of symptomology is its only focus; where it hurts must be where the dysfunction is, right? Wrong.

Picture this: if I grasp a pencil with one hand at each end, pushing my thumbs upward to the sky, the pencil will break in the middle. Traditional healthcare will work on the middle of the pencil. Let's say they repair it with duct tape. If I apply the same force as I did before, it will break again. The middle of the pencil is weak, yes, but the true problem of the pencil is that some clown has his hands on either end of the pencil and keeps pushing his thumbs upward to the sky. *That* is its problem. The eraser isn't breaking off, the lead isn't breaking off—it's the middle that's breaking under the force, but the middle isn't the problem. Now, that's sound logic. And that is using physics: the force is going upward through the center of the pencil, yet addressing what's generating the force is more important than the stability of the pencil to withstand that force.

It's about getting to the root cause. Every Tom, Dick and Harry, claiming to be (to use a buzz word) "holistic," wants to get to the cause—the root cause—of the problem. No, they don't. Nobody gets to the root cause of the problem because we keep treating the symptomology, the sensation of the pain, itself. Those inside the Pain Matrix will keep going to the area—the single area where it hurts and the dysfunction is perceived or assumed to be. They do not see the body as a whole body. They do not treat the physics of the human body as a whole; they only look at the physics of the affected joint. You can't bend your knee? Okay, they say, let's work on all the muscles around that part of the knee that can't bend. You know what? The problem might be somewhere else. It might be the opposite shoulder that's causing all of that, and the knee is just having to react to the shoulder. It's about getting your mind out of single cause, single effect, single solution "logic" and the assumption that where the pain is must be where the problem is located. Those are the two biggest faults I find within the Pain Matrix approach to the treatment of musculoskeletal injuries or dysfunction.

Chapter 4:
Homeostasis
(Nightmares of High School Biology)

Homeostasis: a one-word chapter. Wow, this must be important, huh? It is! Homeostasis is a term we learned in high school biology, and it kind of got beaten into our heads like kettle drums. I remember that many of our test questions, back in the day, used to be fill-in-the-blank. For many of those questions, if I didn't know the answer, I would write in "homeostasis." I figured it would give me a fighting chance, and you know what, it did. It seemed like I got about half of those questions right. It wasn't until I reached my 40s and 50s that I fully realized that homeostasis is, in fact, one of the most important things on this living planet.

We were rather undersold on the importance of homeostasis once we got out of high school biology, but it is huge. To lay it out, your organ problems, back pain, everything—it's about homeostasis. Our organ systems are designed to be at a stable constant. The definition of homeostasis can be more succinctly put by giving you the purpose of a living cell: the only purpose of a living cell is to remain stable. That is the only reason why cells exist. That's why you always hear of cells as being the building blocks of matter. See, you wouldn't build a foundation on unstable ground, right? Well, that's what cells are: they're stable ground. Cells make up tissues, tissues make up organs, and organs make up systems.

Again, we are organ systems and a soul—that's what we are. Therefore, we have to be homeostatic—stable. Our organ systems have to run at stable levels, as you see evidence of in the body with temperature, blood pressure, cholesterol and pH, for instance. Those and other regulations within the body are commonly assessed to determine the condition of the associated organ systems. However, the musculoskeletal system's homeostatic condition is overlooked, even though it, too, must be stable.

What do we mean by "stable?" "Stable" doesn't necessarily involve motion. It doesn't have to move to be stable. In fact, many times, motion is the enemy of stability, and that is part of the reason why we have musculoskeletal problems to begin with. *Musculoskeletal stability is the brain's way of changing our posture and limiting motion so that we don't fall down.* The homeostasis of the musculoskeletal system is regulated by the brain. The brain has an inherent knowledge that goes beyond our conscious mind, beyond what we can reason and rationalize. It merely has inner knowledge that we aren't aware that we have. To explain, the brain will self-preserve and do whatever it must to prevent the body from falling and potentially damaging itself. "Itself," meaning the brain, without consideration of the body. Therefore, it's going to make sure at all times we are stable. If you stand on one leg, you will notice that you slightly bend into the leg that you are standing on, in order to give you a better center of gravity—another physics term. Understand, if you don't have a proper center of gravity, you can fall.

To put it all together, the brain has to make *accommodations* and change your body's *posture* in order to become stable and have a decent center of gravity. That is the role of homeostasis for the musculoskeletal system. The brain needs to make sure that you are stable in all things, including organ health and musculoskeletal health. *It will alter posture and limit motion to make sure that you are stable.* Homeostasis and the musculoskeletal stability of your body, as a whole, is one of the main reasons why we have chronic musculoskeletal pain.

Chapter 5:
How This Works, Short Term

Now that you understand, basically, the role of homeostasis, in terms of the musculoskeletal system and posture, I know you can hardly wait for me to explain how it all works! Right?! How does the brain achieve this homeostatic state? First, let's talk about the brain, itself. Okay, you have a map of your body inside your brain. Think about it: if you want to bend your right elbow, your brain needs to know where to send the signal. If it didn't, your brain would be sending out signals willy-nilly: you'd be kicking your leg out or doing a weird pelvic twist—whatever. So, we know that the brain has to know where to send it, and it absolutely does, by using its map; but your body talks back to your brain, too. If you're bending your right elbow, it says, "Hi, this is the right elbow. Brain, if you bend us any more you might tear ligaments." And the brain is like, "Oh, ok. Sorry. We'll stop." This ability of the body to sense self-movement and body position and communicate that to the brain is called proprioceptive input, or proprioception. See, an injury or an insult to an area can lead to a loss of proprioception from that area. If we feel pain in that location, it does not send the proprioceptive feedback up to the brain. Let's use an example of a baby toe. I stub my right baby toe, and I hit it really hard. My foot is in a lot of pain, and I can feel that pain from the right foot. I consciously know my foot is there; however, the part of the brain that is responsible for movement and weight-bearing and all that good stuff has now lost my right foot. Because of the pain, it cannot receive proprioceptive input from that foot. So, now my brain is in a panic. It thinks, "Oh no! I've lost my right foot!" What is it going to do? I'll tell you exactly what it'll do! *It is going to make an accommodation to that injury.* In the case of my baby toe on my right foot, it's going to roll my ankle in, and I'm going to bear weight on the inside of that foot. Therefore, I don't put any pressure on the baby toe: the pain diminishes, it's back on the map, and the part of my brain that deals with the map can finally find my right foot. It says, "Guys, relax. I have found the foot." Except, there's a problem. If I'm still walking on the inside of my foot, and I am maintaining my normal posture, my center of gravity is off. I have now become unstable. What happens to my posture, as my brain responds, is as follows: my knee angles in, my pelvis on the opposite side shoots out, my low back starts working itself back over to the midline, and the brain elevates the right shoulder. Since I am walking on the inside of my foot, my pelvis height on either side of my spine isn't level, so it's lifting the right shoulder. Finally, my head has to tilt at an angle so that my eyes are kept parallel to the ground. As you can see, for a simple stubbed toe, my brain has made about 8 accommodations to my body—all because I must achieve homeostatic balance and a good center of gravity. My motion will be limited, and my posture will be off, but the brain has ensured that I will not fall. Now, when it makes these changes, you have to realize we have pre-patterned ways of doing things: "synergies," if you will. So, if I want to go and open a door, different muscles have to work at different times and ways to open that door. The brain is not going to issue commands for each and every movement, like: "Biceps, I need you to flex at this angle; supinator muscle, I need you to open the palm 'this many' degrees; brachioradialis, do what you need to do!"—it doesn't give orders on the individual level. It has already pre-planned and figured this out. In the case of opening a door, it's like, "Okay, let's do synergy 42b." Unfortunately, now that my brain has changed my posture by accommodating to the lack of homeostatic balance/instability and thus tightening some muscles and shutting down others, the way my body makes movements also consequently changes; even the way I perform very simple tasks must now be altered because of this accommodation. Anything I do now is going to be altered. If we look at the grand totality of all that's happened, merely from a stubbed baby toe, imagine having to change your entire life and how you do things—everything you do—by hopping on one leg. You might think that is impossible. Well, guess what? Your body goes through that entire change during this and throughout this process with the stubbed toe—not on such a dramatic level, but everything gets altered. Remember earlier when we said the brain doesn't make 100% of its accommodation in one area? It's going to diffuse those changes throughout the body.

Let's talk about the brain limiting motion. How the brain limits that motion is twofold: it's going to utilize muscle spasms and inflammation. See, inflammation is like pouring bleach on an open wound: it hurts. But it's also like Styrofoam peanuts for packing. We've probably all had injuries where something has swollen and can't move. Well, it's that inflammation in there limiting the motion within the joint. Remember also that muscles are the force that attaches to bones, which are levers, which move the joints. So, if the muscles are tightened up, the joint cannot freely move. This is how the brain is making that homeostatic change to limit motion: the brain will tighten a muscle, and it uses another part of the mid-brain called the basal ganglia, then, to inhibit motion. If you ever look at somebody who has their shoulders rolled in forward, their pectoralis (or "pec") muscles, which go from the chest and attach to the ball-and-socket joint of the shoulders, tighten up, pulling the shoulders in. However, you never see people walking down the street with their shoulders going back, then forward, then back, then forward, in a dramatic fashion—no. The brain will tighten the muscle, and it will shut that down via the basal ganglia. What then happens to the work load? Remember, Einstein taught us it cannot be destroyed. That work, which is a form of energy, has to go somewhere else; therefore, more workload is placed upon the biceps and deltoids. Along with limiting the motion with the muscles, the brain also has to change joint angles. Remember how I said my ankle is going to roll in? Well, that is a change in the joint angle at the ankle. And I said that the knee would also bend in? That is a change of the joint angle at the knee. So, how will the brain to do it? Well, it's like a pulley system. It's going to tighten one muscle in one area and make another one not exert as much energy; so, one side will pull down harder than the other, and that changes the angle of the joint. In addition, it will tighten the other muscle up to make sure it's stable. The brain will go around limiting motion while changing joint angles and dumping in inflammation. This is the nature of accommodations; this is how the brain maintains its homeostatic control. Always remember it's about stability—it's about homeostasis. The brain's response to any kind of insult, injury or trauma is to maintain homeostatic control for the body. The brain could not care less if you can move or move properly; and, frankly, the brain does not care at all if you hurt. As long as you are stable, the brain is happy because you are in homeostasis.

Chapter 6:

How This Works, Long Term

In the previous chapter, we talked about how the brain's desire to keep our musculoskeletal system in homeostatic control leads to accommodations—tightening up of muscles and inflammation, etc. How long do these accommodations last? The answer is *forever*. Stepping briefly back inside the Pain Matrix, standard healthcare has wrongly assumed that once an injury resolves itself, the accommodation will go away. Well, the truth is, it doesn't. You see, the last time the brain was normal for that area, it lost that area. Referring back to the stubbed toe example, the last time my brain let me stand on my foot correctly, my foot felt pain, and it lost proprioception—it lost my foot. I was unstable. So, the brain is not motivated to change anything back. It's in a homeostatic condition. It made it to homeostasis; therefore, why should it change back? *Remember, change is the opposite of stable*. The brain doesn't change just because. It doesn't change posture to make the musculoskeletal system better; it always changes the musculoskeletal system to keep it stable. That's the only time the brain will change it. No change is good change, as long as we are stable. Realize, we go through life stacking accommodations one upon another, upon another, upon another—*and the brain never undoes them*. Take a look at a 5-year-old standing straight up, compared to a 75-year-old standing up. If that doesn't prove my point, I don't know what would! What happens is that these accommodations, sooner or later, will cause the affected areas of the body to give out. Remember your physics lesson with the pencil? Excessive forces applied at wrong angles leads to the consequent breakage: friction, deterioration, muscle injury and so on. See, it might not be that disc from 20 years ago that is causing your friend the pain. It could be the accommodation in and around that area that is causing that pain. If you recall, tissue on the inside of the body heals at about the same rate as tissue on the outside of the body. No one cuts their hand and bleeds for 20 years—I know I haven't. So, to blame a disc—rounding up the usual suspects—is an old-fashioned, outdated mode of thinking perpetuated by the Pain Matrix. However, what we can recognize is that the accommodation that the brain made 20 years ago to that disc is still going to be there, and that's why the pain is in the same area. Each and every one of these accommodations stack up, and it leads to poorer posture; it keeps worsening, and it leads to even more improper movement. Just because you are "old" doesn't mean you can't be flexible! Those within the Pain Matrix look at accommodations as a temporary event. It's actually a lifelong process. When we get older, there are certain realities to our bodies. Our ligaments aren't as taut. Muscles have to tighten up to secure the joint a little bit, but not to the extent that we have people all hunched over, living every minute of their life in pain. No! That comes from longevity—not the longevity of the person—the longevity of the accommodation. Standard healthcare is quick to give out diagnoses of arthritis. Well, it's good old "Uncle Arthur." If you want to hit my hot button, talk about "Uncle Arthur." Here is something that people don't realize and don't think about hard enough: there is no device in mankind that can objectively measure pain. I can't hook something up to you and tell you that you are reading a 7.2 on my trusty pain-o-meter. No, we don't do it and can't do it. It's all subjective. As a result, we don't know where the origins of pain are. We are as inept at deducing pain and the science of pain as a 5-year-old is at calculus. I know that sounds pretty harsh, but it's true. One of the things people don't realize is how much healthcare really doesn't know. For some reason, the provider tells you the problem is arthritis and that you're going to have to live with it, and it's accepted as truth. People follow the expert's diagnosis and go on anti-inflammatories, they limit what they do, and they pine for what they used to be able to do. Again, we go back to the single cause, single effect, because healthcare does not know the origins of pain and how it works, precisely, and what could be causing the pain. They are quick to find a single cause. If you have any degeneration in a joint, they will call it "arthritis" and tell you that is where your pain is coming from. But is it? Is 100% of that pain all due to that little tiny spur there? Here's the secret: they don't know. They are going to act like they know, but they don't. No one knows. Maybe only 10% of that pain is caused by that little tiny spur. So many times in my practice, I have seen what I call the "death diagnosis." It's not a morbidity diagnosis; it's a diagnosis of, "you have arthritis, and you are going to have to live with it," and that person now is condemned to a life of inactivity with pain. The provider doesn't know! They are assuming! They have to find that single cause for that single effect. Gladly, what I see with those types of people who come into my office is that their pain level goes down dramatically when I address the accommodations that the brain made due to old injuries. It is the ability to get the brain to undo those accommodations, which will allow freedom of movement. With proper movement comes a dissipation of pain. As long as we are stuck in a posture riddled with accommodations, we will always have improper movement, generating pain. I frequently use this example: I can't tell you how many times I hear about a 70ish-year-old woman getting rotator cuff surgery. Now, this woman has never pitched a day of major league baseball in her life. She doesn't lift heavy weights; if anything, her activities have been limited. So, why did she blow out a rotator cuff? Because of poor posture, created by accommodations to previous injuries. It's not because of her age! It's that she has carried these accommodations around for years, and the rotator cuff finally gave out. That's why she needs surgery. I am not saying surgeries are never needed, but why can't we stop this process well before it ever gets to this point? That is what the Vibrate-A-Way™ system does: it addresses the accommodations the brain makes to our posture to maintain homeostasis—in a word, stability.

Chapter 7:
Now the Solution:
The Future of Pain Relief

So far, I have described overall how the brain will make accommodative changes in response to pain. We're talking about pain felt in a joint or in a muscle. These accommodative changes that the brain makes last forever: the brain will not undo them, for the reason being that the brain needs to remain in homeostasis. So, you pose the obvious, logical question of, "Ok, so these changes in my posture are the problem, and they won't self-correct; do you have the solution?"

The solution I present to you is our revolutionary Vibrate-A-Way™ system: we are actually going to communicate to your brain via your proprioceptive nerve endings, with the purpose of undoing those accommodations to your posture and, thus, movement. Remember, proprioception is how the body talks back to the brain. They communicate through your hundreds of millions of proprioceptive nerve endings: those nerve endings are located in your muscles, your skin, your joints, and they basically tell your brain where you are in time and space and how you are moving. Now, people who want to split hairs will say kinesthesia is about movement, and proprioception is about standard; but you can lump them all together under the umbrella of proprioception. It's because of proprioception that you don't fall down when you are on a boat out on a lake. As the waves rock the boat, you automatically lean your body from one side to the other to avoid falling over. Well, that is your proprioceptive nervous system in action. Your brain will again make these changes to your posture to ensure your stability as the boat rolls from one side to the other.

In the Vibrate-A-Way™ program, we are going to utilize these nerves in your body to talk to the brain. These proprioceptive nerve endings respond to different stimuli: they will respond to vibration, percussion, pressure, stretch, velocity and angulations. All these different things trigger a response from the brain. It is the classic feedback system, sort of like a thermostat: when the thermostat "senses" that the room is colder than 68 degrees, it will kick on the furnace, which warms the room to 68 degrees and automatically stops. Likewise, the proprioceptive nerve endings give feedback to a signal: the brain initiates movement or a posture, and the proprioceptive nervous system gives a feedback; based on that, the brain alters the original posture or movement. That is precisely what we are influencing: this control loop system. We are going to utilize vibration to basically talk to your brain to get the brain to make changes to the accommodations. *Because the brain is what created the accommodations in the first place, no matter what you do, it must be the brain which returns everything back to how and where it was and should be.* I can stretch a muscle as much as I like, but if my brain wants that muscle tightened, it will tighten it. I can stretch my "pec" muscles by doing a door stretch to try to get my shoulders to come back, but guess what? They always roll forward again. Why? Because that is where the brain wants them to be for its proprioceptive stability, whether that posture is correct or not. As we're basically going around, applying vibration to different areas of the body, it will be like turning on and off feedback switches to the brain. Based on that feedback, the brain will then make changes to the accommodations. **So, it's kind of like untangling all the things that the brain did, while making it the brain's idea to undo them.**

We apply the vibration in a systemic pattern—a sequential pattern. We have always heard that the brain is like a computer; well, it is. I know I'm going old-school—and a lot of you readers might laugh at how old-school I am—but I will use an example of binary code. If I was programming by entering binary code as input and got a "1" and a "0" mixed up—even if I had a million ones and zeros in this code—it wouldn't work. That is why the brain is very particular about the sequence and pattern of vibration. Many times, people apply vibration to where it hurts, and—as I pointed out earlier—where you hurt generally isn't the problem: the dysfunction is on the side that *doesn't* hurt. By applying vibration in this specific pattern, it will unlock the postural deviations that the brain had made.

Proper posture means proper movement, which means an absence of pain. When we perform the Vibrate-A-Way™ system, people feel better! They can move! But wait: there is a problem, and that problem is homeostasis. Ugh—here we go again, back to homeostasis. If you recall, the brain couldn't care less if you can move better or if you hurt or not: it wants to make sure you are stable. Therefore, in the beginning, the brain is like, "Oh yeah, this feels really good." But, you start to do something—you drive a distance, you go back to work, you do something around the house—and the brain is like, "No, no. We do it like this, where we are stable." So, the brain takes your posture back to how it's had it. What that does, is actually force me to *use homeostasis against the brain*. It's sort of like the old adage to "fight fire with fire." Now, I am not a big fan of that—I always thought you fought fire with water or extinguishers, but you know what? In this case, it is spot on. So, how we're going to use homeostasis against the brain is like this: I created a system in which we apply the vibrational protocols again and reset that posture to where we want it. Of course, later but probably sooner (at this point), you are going to apply some kind of stimulus by doing something where the brain will respond by bringing it all back again to where it currently identifies as stable. However, don't be discouraged: we are going to go back and forth so many times that, all of a sudden, what used to be homeostatic—what used to be stable to the brain—is no longer stable. Now we have the brain right where we want it! See, the brain is lazy. Depending on what you read and whom you ask, some say that the brain is composed of 80% water; one of the characteristics of water is that it takes the path of least resistance. The brain has proven in study after study that it does that. It takes the path of least resistance. So, instead of recreating a whole new posture with a bunch of different accommodations, the brain is simply going to accept the one that this system gives it, which is the unaltered posture that you had before it started stacking accommodation upon accommodation.

That is how that works, and it takes repetition. That's why Vibrate-A-Way™ is a 60-day program. People ask, "Why does it take 60 days?" I don't know. It just does. I have been doing this for about 10 years, and that is the pattern I have found. After about 60 days, the brain gives up on trying to go back to the old posture. The technique, the Vibrate-A-Way™ system, takes roughly 20 minutes to do. During those 60 days, receiving the protocols too often is rare; but the frequency does vary by individual. Some people need it to be performed 5 days a week, but others need it 3 days a week or even just once a week. I find that it is safer to err on the side of having it performed too often because, one, the technique feels good—it really does feel good. And it's very uncommon to overdo it—after all, we are getting the brain to reset your posture. But 20 minutes a day, at least 3 to 5 times a week, for 60 days will dramatically improve posture and movement. During that time, you always want to do what you normally do. If you normally work out lifting weights, keep doing it. If you walk 5 miles a day, keep doing it. If you crochet, keep doing it. Any fool can make you feel better by telling you not to do something, then once the pain goes away and you start to do that activity again—you hurt. We need to correct the posture based on what you do. Remember talking about the synergies? About how your brain has patterns and programs for how to do things? Well, the more you can do as we correct the old posture during the use of those synergies, the quicker the brain will make global changes and start to only use correct posture and movement with everything. Furthermore, there is a break-even point when the brain starts to see where this is going. Even with a new stimulus, it will retain this corrected posture and identify it as its new "stable." Again, the brain is taking the path of least resistance.

If you've made the choice to escape the Pain Matrix, you now have the solution, the future of pain relief: the Vibrate-A-Way™ system. By following this system, doing the technique for these roughly 60 days, you'll peel away the accommodative layers and reset your brain to maintain homeostasis using correct posture for its stability with correct movements. With your posture and movements as they should be, you'll enjoy relief from the pain and get on with your life!

Chapter 8:
The Nuts and Bolts

In the previous chapters, I have taken you through the old patterns of the Pain Matrix followed by standard healthcare and the general population today. I've shared with you the reasons I felt compelled to search for a New System—both a new System of *viewing* the problem and a new System of *correcting* the problem.

The old way of thinking is "single cause, single effect, single solution" and "the side/joint/area that is symptomatic is the problem or where the dysfunction is." The New System of viewing a musculoskeletal problem is that the body is one continuous unit and that the physics of the machine that we call the human body requires an overall look at the *entire* machine—everything is connected. The New System shows us that, in many cases, the side that hurts is actually the side that is working—and it's working too hard. The side that *isn't* working is the problem because all the work that it *used* to do is now being shifted over to other areas. Of course, this doesn't mean that if you roll your ankle and tear your ligaments, the sprained ankle is not the problem, and it's got to be the other side—no, not at all. I am talking chronic long-term pain. And the reason is, with chronic long-term pain, your brain accommodates to injuries and dysfunctions and repetitive use/motion (think sitting at a desk for long periods). It accommodates throughout the entire body, making changes on a global scale. Remember, the problems are global, and the accommodation will be global.

The other thing we know is that once the injury or the problem resolves, the brain doesn't undo the accommodation. It is there forever, unless you tell the brain to stop it, and that is the other bite of knowledge we need to take from the New System: no matter what medication, no matter what stretches, no matter how many manipulations you get, nothing will change that accommodation. The only thing that will change that accommodation is the brain which gave you the accommodation. The brain is the master computer. By applying vibration in a sequential pattern throughout the body—it took me years of experimentation and research to decipher this code—we can talk to the brain via the proprioceptive nervous system and tell the brain to undo those postural accommodations.

So, with that in mind, let's go ahead and start taking a look at how you can find your postural deviations and how you can apply the Vibrate-A-Way™ system to your body to improve your posture and movement.

Chapter 9:
Making Vibrate-A-Way™ Work for You

When a person comes to my clinic to address an issue they have, I make it very clear that I do not treat conditions. The complaint might be a bad back or a sore knee, and the desired end result of their treatment is improvement. Keeping true to my philosophy, the first thing I focus on is their entire posture and then movement. You see, I know that if I improve a person's posture, I can improve their motion. And if their motion improves, most of the time, their pain in the area of complaint will go away.

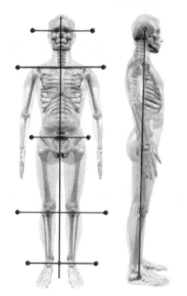

So, how's *your* posture? The first jumping-off point we should have now, moving forward, is to look at what your posture is doing. Here's what you'll need to do: get out your cell phone or camera. We are going to take a couple of pictures: the first is from the front, and the other is from the side. It's best to have someone take these pictures, so you can stand with your arms at your side and look straight ahead. On most phones or tablets, you can draw on the picture digitally, but I am old-school and like to have a copy in my hands. So, I always recommend that you print the pictures, and when you have those pictures in front of you, you might be able to see the deviations in posture without even drawing any lines to help guide yourself. That is quite common. Regardless, we are still going to draw the lines:

- The first line you'll draw will be the front view of your center of gravity. Take the front-to-back picture and a ruler to measure the distance between the feet. It doesn't matter what frame of reference you use—the two big toes, the middle of each foot, the shoelaces—your reference point is irrelevant. Just measure the distance between the two feet, and the halfway point is going to be where we start our line. From that halfway point between the 2 feet, draw a straight line (parallel to the side margins of your picture) up your body, right through the top of your head.
- Next, put a dot on the center of each eye and connect the dots with a line.
- After that, you are going to draw a dot on the top of each shoulder and, again, connect those two dots with a straight line across.
- Then, on the front of the arm, at the spot where the elbow bends, you are going to put a dot there and connect those dots.
- On the top of your pelvis—the crest—you are going to again put a dot and connect each dot with a line (this is commonly called the "hip bones" on each side).
- Finally, right on the center of each kneecap, draw a dot and a line connecting those.

Here is what you should look for:

- Half of your body should fall to the left of the line, and the other half should fall to the right
- Deviations in which more of your body is off to one side or the other indicate that your center of gravity is off
- Are your eyes level? If not, your head could be tilted, and muscles in the neck could be pulling it one way or another
- Are the shoulders and elbows on the same plane, or is one side higher than the other?
- Is one side of the pelvis higher than the other (are the "hip bones" even)?
- Are your knees level?

After you have made the observations, set that photo off to the side. Next, we are going to look at the side view of your center of gravity.

- First, you are going to find the ankle bone—the little round protrusion at the ankle. Draw a dot right on that protrusion and continue that line straight upwards, again, through the top of the head. The line is parallel to the side margins of the photo.
- The line should go through certain landmarks: one is the knee but not necessarily the middle—just slightly backwards of what is the center of the knee.
- Next is the ball-and-socket of the hip joint, and if you are wondering how to tell, honestly, it should go through the very center of the buttocks—the area we associate with the hip and the pelvis.
- The line should go through the center of your shoulder and up into your ear—right up through it.

Let's make some observations of the side view:

- Is your body, as a whole, leaning forward or backward of your center line of gravity?
- Are your knees forward or backward of the line?
- Is your head tilted forward or backward? Where are your ears in relation to the line?

Remember that the straight line up-and-down is your center of gravity. If you have any deviation, this is going to create issues in movement. As I have told you before, good posture leads to good movement. Poor posture leads to poor movement. As I beat this dead horse—what does that mean? Poor posture means pain. Dysfunction: it happens because of that poor motion. So, when we have these deviations from the postural norms, both front-to-back and sideways, usually, what we see is that one or a group of muscles have worked together to be tightened, and then the brain shuts those down. In other instances, there are muscles that just are flaccid: they are not up to tone, and they are not working properly. A third cause is one or a group of these muscles are tight and *overworking*. So, we have "tight and shut down," we have "basically stretched out and not working," and we have "tight and overworking." These 3 categories are how the brain works out its physics—how it changes our posture and movement—by manipulating how the muscles express themselves in the length and tone that they have. Normally, a combination of all 3 of these will apply, not just one or the other.

Now that you have observed your own posture, let me tell you about some of the most common postural deviations that I see, and you can check if any number of these apply to you.

1. The head is forward of the midline
2. The shoulders are rolled in
3. One shoulder is higher than the other
4. The pelvis is rolled forward (the pelvis is forward of the knees and ankles)
5. Increased lumbar curve (Commonly called swayback)
6. Lack of lumbar curve (Straight line in the lumbar spine)

Now that we've identified these common postural deviations, let's talk about what causes them. The first is the head-forward posture. This is going to be caused by a tightening of the forward flexion muscles of the neck and shoulders. That means that the neck muscles that contract to allow you to tuck in your chin or bow your head are tightening. If you run the midline of the throat (at your Adam's apple) and move out sideways slightly and push in, you can feel where those muscles are tight and tender. In addition, the brain inhibits or weakens the extension muscles—the muscles in the back of the neck that pull the head up. That way, the brain can alter your center of gravity by having the head forward. You see, the head and the shoulders go together. A lot of the shoulder muscles connect to the neck and vice-versa. So, if your head is forward, your shoulders are going to most likely roll forward. We're actually talking about several muscle groups being tightened: shoulder muscles, chest muscles, and even abdominal muscles. Your "pec" muscles are the big muscles that roll your shoulders in, and then what happens is that the brain will also inhibit and weaken the shoulder and back muscles that pull the shoulders back. So, that is why we get the rolled-in shoulders and the head forward. I call it the "Fred Flintstone" posture. If you have ever watched the "Flintstones" cartoons, you can see that is

Fred's problem right there: his head is forward, and his shoulders are rolled in as he stomps in wanting his dinner!

One shoulder being higher than another can be caused by the tightening of the shoulder. You know the upper "trap" muscles—those muscles that when someone comes up behind you and starts squeezing around your shoulders you melt like butter? Well, those are the upper trapezius muscles. The muscles around your scapula, which is your shoulder blade, become tightened, and the brain will inhibit and weaken the extension muscles, or the muscles that pull the shoulder back. That will usually involve the lower trapezius and the "lats"—the latissimus dorsi.

If your pelvis is rolled forward, your hip flexors, your "quads" and your stomach muscles are all going to be tightened; your gluteal and hamstring muscles will be inhibited. That way, the pelvis can be pulled forward.

And, of course, if you have an increased lumbar curve, obviously, the muscles in the back are going to be way tightened. In the case of the decreased curve—the straight back—again, your core muscles will be weakened.

When we look at the posture front-to-back and sideways, we want to look for these things. How has the body been altered from textbook normal? Textbook normal is basically common sense. Are you a straight line? Does the line go from your ankle up through your ears, and is everything else right in the middle? Front-to-back—does the line reach from the center in between your feet and extend straight up, right through your nose and in between your eyes? If so, then that is good. It's just common sense. There is no big mystery or complicated science behind it. So, find your postural deviations and keep these pictures because these are going to be the beginning. As you progress utilizing the Vibrate-A-Way™ System, you will be able to measure your progress by taking updated photos and drawing those same exact lines. You may wish to take a "before" analysis and another analysis every 15 days, so about every quarter of the 60 days of the program. Feel good about the improvements you're making!

Chapter 10:
Measuring Your Motion

The next component to observe is, naturally, motion. How do you move? The easiest way to do this is to set up your phone or camera and record yourself walking. Make sure that you record yourself walking in a straight line to the camera and away from the camera. Now you will be able to review your motion and your movement. Walking is the simplest of movements, and it is the action that we do the most. In that, the body can reveal many of the secrets of what the brain has done to it. Let's take a look at your walking in a big-picture frame of mind. We are not going to break this down and make it into a meticulous scientific approach here. We are just going to look at big-picture—the things that you can see, what is apparent.

When I analyze a person's gait, the feet are what I observe first. Our normal gait cycle, made simple, is that we hit the ground with our heel, the foot flattens out, and then it pushes off as the other leg is doing the same thing (ultra-simply put, "**heel strike, foot flat, toe off**"). It goes back and forth in this way. Any deviation from that cycle tells me that we have an altered posture that, again, is changing the physics. The most common alterations to the posture that affect movement are 1) a rolled forward pelvis, 2) the tailbone being out posterior (going backwards), or 3) your calves and hamstrings are very tight. With any of these three, we find that you do not get that full expression of the heel striking, the foot going flat, and then toeing off.

The next thing we want to observe is the pelvis. How does a pelvis move? When we walk, we have something that I like to refer to as a "pelvic rhythm." As we take a step, we bear weight on one side, on one leg, as the other swings through. Therefore, the pelvis will slightly shift up on the leg that is swinging, and it will go down on the leg that is bearing the weight. This leg swing is actually caused mostly by the pelvis. The official term is the sacroiliac joint, which we have probably all heard of that at some point. Our pelvis movement comes from the sacroiliac joint, and the majority of the leg swing in our walking comes from that sacroiliac joint and pelvis movement. Here is a quick little exercise to do with your hands. With your left hand make a "C" and with your right hand make a reverse "C"; hold them about 2 inches apart. Now, without moving any other part of your arm, just your wrist, move your right hand back at the wrist towards you, towards your body. And then with the left hand, do the opposite and alternate your "Cs" forward and backward. So, if one goes up, the other goes down: that is how the pelvis moves when we walk. Do you see the rotation? What I look for when watching someone's gait is the movement in their buttocks—that's where the pelvis is. I look to see if, as it rotates in and out, the leg that bears the weight goes downward at the pelvis, and the swinging leg goes up a little bit. Essentially, is the walking movement mimicking the exercise with the "C"?

I look for that pelvic rhythm while they are walking, or I notice if there is a kind of improper side-to-side rotation at the pelvis. Let's take our hands again and make the same "Cs": this time, instead of *twisting* our wrists to make our "Cs" alternately move forward and backward, we are going to *bend* our wrists alternately. Your

"Cs" will consequently move side-to-side and that is what the pelvis is doing. Again, that is improper motion.

Another deviation from the "pelvic rhythm" that I see in walking is that one side of the pelvis is up high (and stays high) and creates a kind of teeter-totter, side-to-side walk. The pelvis doesn't do its normal rotation back-and-forth but it actually goes side-to-side, or one leg hangs up higher on one side.

When we walk, the pelvic rotation is critical for our leg swing. If our leg swings normally, it is like a pendulum—straight forward. When the foot lands, it's just a slight toe-out, as our feet are never perfectly pointing with toes straight forward: they are slightly off—they slightly rotate outwards. Sometimes, when observing the leg swing, I notice that the person is just kind of swinging the whole pelvis side-to-side, and the feet are pointing abnormally outward.

The upper trunk is next to observe. Are the shoulders and the upper trunk forward of the pelvis? If so, the weight is being carried forward of the center of gravity, and that is going to limit motion on the pelvis.

When observing gait, I also listen. That's right: I can hear when someone has an abnormal gait—when their pelvis is moving side-to-side, one side is higher than the other, or the upper trunk is forward of the midline. I hear a very heavy walk: thump, thump, thump. Do you know a heavy walker in your life? Usually, we do if we live in an apartment and have people living on the floor above us! Well, that heavy walking is a result of an improper center of gravity during motion. When listening to gait, I also sometimes hear a scuffle step like the shuffling of feet. You can hear that friction on the carpet, on the floor, on the ground. Well, that scuffling step is an indication that they are not getting clearance on their leg swing—that, again, their posture is off, and it's affecting their motion and their movement.

Another thing that I commonly see is that a person will short-step. We all have a stride length. Now, you could measure it and say it should be "x" amount of inches, but every body's stride length is different. There really is no set standard when you take into account a person's leg length. So, what I want to look at is just common sense. For that person's size and leg length, does it look like they are taking a normal stride? Or does it look short? If I see somebody with a short stride, then I realize that the brain is trying to make them stable and is limiting their motion on that stride. It wants to make sure that they won't fall forward. The main thing that correlates to that short stride when someone walks is the fact that they're forward of their center of gravity. If they're forward of their center of gravity so their upper trunk is forward of that midline (remember the analysis that we did on your posture), we're going to see that the brain will limit motion.

So, that is how we analyze gait, and you can go through everything I just told you and simplify it even more:

- Is the person straight up and down?
- Do the legs look like they are moving normally?
- Do the feet generally point straight ahead?
- Do they go "heel strike, foot flat, toe off" when they walk?
- Are their shoulders back?

That's all it really is. If you have deviated from any of that, then you know the brain has made changes.

When I review a video of patients and show them their gait, it's kind of entertaining for me because generally the first phrase I hear out of their mouth is, "Oh my goodness! Is that how I really walk?" And half, if not more, want to try it again. They want to improve it. They want to show me that they could do better. And you know what? Those alterations in movement still remain. See, **one of the biggest fallacies we believe is that we can consciously improve our posture or our movement**. And here's why. We can stand straighter if we think about it. We can get better range of motion if we work on stretching it or do other exercises to get more motion. But the fact remains that the brain has changed the posture internally. It has altered the expression of muscles. We might stand straighter, but we're using the wrong muscles to do that work. We might be able to lift our arm higher than we had been, but we're using the wrong muscles to do it. We are now using muscles which main priority or purpose is not to lift that arm but to do something else. So, in essence, we are putting more of a work demand on muscles that shouldn't have that work demand placed upon them. Bottom line is we're making it worse. I know this is going to sound strong, but I am a blunt person, so here it is: I want to vomit every time I see those ads, "Improve your posture with this home exercise!" Do this. Buy this contraption. Improve your posture by being more mindful. It doesn't work. You're being sold a bill of goods, and at what cost to your muscles and joints? Maybe there is some improvement, but again, it is improvement made to an already-altered posture and movement system caused by the brain to keep you stable.

From now on, when we think about movement, let's start to view movement how it is correctly and normally. It's not about whether or not you get the job done, it's actually *how* you get the job done. When it comes to human movement, it's more about the style points than it is anything else.

So, let's take a look at joint-specific motion and whether or not that's been altered. Of course, with the posture, we know that our head and neck should be erect. The head's not tilted or bent forward or to one side or the other. How you can also tell during motion whether that area's been affected is—first off—rotate your head to the left and to the right. For most people, that range of motion is going to be limited, but you know what? To me, the reduced range of motion is not the important point: *the important point is what muscles are doing what*. So, if you have somebody near you, ask for their help, or you can even do it for yourself: turn your neck to the left. What muscle is tightening up? See, all motion should be smooth. The muscles should do the work and not have this sudden, very expressive grab. So, as you turn your head to the left, do you notice on the right side that maybe a muscle is just getting really tight? Or you feel a muscle tugging really hard on the left side as you turn to the left? Then turn to the right and make the same observations. What are you feeling? Does it feel smooth, or do you feel that hard tug? Try another one. When you bend your head forward, do you feel the muscles in the back of your neck getting very tight, trying to almost prevent you from doing it? Do you notice the muscles on the side of your neck that kind of connect from the bottom of your ear down toward your shoulder? Are they tight? Every motion you have should be smooth. One of the phrases I use in my clinic when I am working on patients is, "I want to make sure that all the muscles that should be working, are, and all the ones that shouldn't, don't." That's the bottom line of what we are doing here. And you don't have to know anatomy. You can buy my more advanced book or become certified to perform the Vibrate-A-Way™ system to learn that anatomy and how it goes, but for right now just to do this at home. It's common sense. Do the muscles have an abnormal tug expression when you move your head left and right, back, down and up?

Let's move on to the shoulder—shoulder motion. First off, just move your shoulder/arm all around in different degrees of motion. Hold your arm in front of you and lift it forward and up like you are raising your hand to answer a question. Take it out to the side and lift it as high as you can out to the side. Take it backwards behind you. Straighten your arm and move it over across your body, and then take that straight arm and go as far back as you can. Do you feel any abnormal tugs? Or, does the person helping you feel that when you try these motions? Feel around the entire shoulder as you do this. One of the catch-all tests that I do to determine correct shoulder motion is the collarbone test: when you raise your arm straight up in the air in front of you like you are answering a question, there is a specific pattern of motion that happens. The shoulder blade rotates down and in. It spins, and that pops the ball-and-socket joint up in the air—but the collarbone (or clavicle) connects to the shoulder blade. That is the acromioclavicular joint, so if you ever watch a sporting event and you hear the "AC joint," that is what they are talking about. If the shoulder blade is going to spin, then the collarbone naturally has to spin. I test for that, and so should you.

What you are going to do is have somebody stand behind you and put their finger (with moderate-to-light pressure) on the muscle right behind the collar bone. They are barely going to touch the back end of that collarbone. What's going to happen is the person is going to leave their finger there while you lift your arm straight up in the air in front of you like you are answering a question. The person who is applying the pressure should feel that collarbone spin and push back on his finger. If so, then you know that you have correct shoulder motion. If that mechanism isn't working properly, then I can guarantee you that all those other motions that you have done with your arm and shoulder are not working properly, either. Here is why: most times, if that collarbone doesn't spin, then you'll find that your shoulders will also be rolled in. The "pec" muscle (the pectoralis muscle) goes from the breastbone (the sternum) out to the ball-and-socket. So, if that shoulder is rolled in, then we know that the "pec" muscle is tight. But the "pec" muscle also connects to the collarbone. Therefore, if the "pec" muscle is tight enough to roll a shoulder in, it's going to be so tight that it won't allow the collarbone to spin. If the collarbone can't spin, then your shoulder blade can't spin; if your shoulder blade can't spin, you have to lift your arm in a different and abnormal way. That's the true reason why most people feel tightness in their upper "trap"—you know, from your neck to your shoulders—but everybody wants to blame it on stress. Even healthcare practitioners will say, "Wow, these are tight! You must be stressed!" Well, bull-hockey. Stress is the 2-gallon can of gasoline that I am pouring on a bonfire. It doesn't help it, but it certainly isn't the cause of it. You see, when our shoulder motion isn't proper, when we lift our arm straight up in the air, that upper "trap" muscle now has to elevate the shoulder blade more than what it should. So, that way, it creates an angle for the shoulder blade to allow that ball-and-socket joint to go up. Then it gives an angle so that the retractor muscles of the shoulder (that are located in the back) now have to lift the arm up, and that's not their job; it's an altered motion caused by altered posture. And that's why that collarbone test is so determining: we have to find out the most important point of what muscles are doing what.

For elbows and wrists, it's the same thing. Try moving them in all the different planes of motion that you can. Do you feel extra tightness? If you try to pull your wrist back, is it limited in motion? If so, press on the top of the forearm and feel those muscles. All the muscles that pull the hand backwards are located on the top of the forearm. If you do the opposite motion and bend your wrist in like you're going to do a bicep curl, is that motion limited? If so, the muscles on the other (under) side of that forearm are tight. The brain is limiting motion.

A major one to test is the low back. Bend forwards, bend backwards, and side-to-side. Are you feeling tightness in any region when you do this? Is the abdomen tight? Are your hip flexors tight, or your "quads"? Is something moving abnormally? Is something creating too much expression?

One of the main muscles that the brain will tighten up and shut down are the hamstrings. When the brain rolls the pelvis forward, it needs to *keep* the pelvis forward. In order to do that, it's going to shorten the hip flexors and shut them down. That way, that hip flexor is always pulling the pelvis forward; it's going to stretch out the hamstring and tighten it. To create a visual, you kind of have a rope on one end and a rope on the other: one is shorter than the other, and the other has to go longer. That's why hamstrings are really weak. It's not because we don't pay enough attention in the gym: it's the fact that the brain is using them to secure the pelvis, and it has to first lengthen them then tighten them. Are your hamstrings tight? Lie down on your stomach. Have someone you know push down on your hamstrings. First off, you will feel it. Second off, they will, too.

Check the knee. Does your knee motion feel stiff? Does it feel tight? If so, then we notice that we have imbalances in the hamstrings, the "quads", the calves, and a muscle group called the anterior compartment—located on the outside of your shin. On the very inside of your shin, there's nothing there but bone and skin; but on the outside, you can feel that muscle. Well, those muscles tighten up, too.

It's this entire combination that prevents that "heel strike, foot flat, toe off" when you walk; therefore, you want to be sure to observe and note all the different motions while feeling for abnormal muscle expression. All the right muscles should be working, and all the wrong muscles shouldn't: they should be doing their own job and not another one's job. You don't have to possess an extensive knowledge of anatomy to figure this out. It's simple. Just move and put your hand on the muscles that move. Does the muscle and motion feel normal and smooth? If you apply a little bit of pressure while it's moving, is it sore? That's the simplest home self-test you can do: as you are moving, put just firm pressure on the involved muscles—not a death grip—and then move the joint. You can feel those muscles moving. Does it hurt? Does it feel like one is really going crazy? That will give you an indication.

With the knowledge of where your posture is not correct and what motion has abnormal muscle expression, you are better able to see how your accommodations are affecting you. Remember, all these changes that have happened to your posture and your motion have happened because the brain is trying to make your musculoskeletal system stable. As you feel the abnormal muscle expression, perhaps now you can understand why muscles wear out, why we have long-term chronic pain. Perhaps now, you can understand why, if a muscle does a wrong job and is working too hard, you are more susceptible to injury. Can you now see that when your posture, motion and your muscle expression are all altered, it's more important about *how* you do something than what you do? It helps to take away the mystery of "I don't know. I didn't do anything." You know what? Based on that poor posture and that muscle expression, perhaps now you can see how you were *just ready* to have something happen.

Chapter 11:
Applying the Vibrate-A-Way™ System

Ok, so let's recap before we progress to the next episode! We've established the existence of the Pain Matrix, along with some of its attributes and ways it's maintained. We've realized that the "single cause, single effect, single solution" system of the Pain Matrix is designed, whether intentionally or not, to keep us trapped within the Pain Matrix for its own survival and offers no true solution to chronic musculoskeletal pain and dysfunction. We've learned that there's a New System on the rise to revolutionize the Pain Matrix and finally offer a solution—a true solution—to this pain and dysfunction: the Vibrate-A-Way™ System! We've also recognized how the brain utilizes homeostasis to make changes and accommodations to our body based on previous trauma, repetitive use or motion, whatever it might be. Most recently, we have also learned how to look at our body to see those alterations or changes in our posture and in our motion. But now comes the time when we learn how to apply the Vibrate-A-Way™ System!

It's time to talk about the utilization of vibration to make the brain change our posture. Do you recall talking about the proprioceptive nerves? Those are the nerves that tell the brain where our body is in time and space. Stimulating those nerves through vibration will cause the brain to change the posture based on that feedback.

Let's get to the nuts and bolts of the application of the vibration. We first must establish the fact that **the purpose of this vibration is not to relax the muscles**. Many people have said to me, "Oh yeah, I have a home massager that vibrates. I do this therapy at home." No, they don't. Generally, what they do is to apply the vibration to the area that is sore, and they will leave it on there for 10 to 15 minutes. Now, don't get me wrong: there is some therapeutic value to that. It increases blood flow, and it gives some palliative care. In stark contrast, what Vibrate-A-Way™ does is utilize a specific pattern and sequence of a vibrational stimulus to the proprioceptive nerves, which then causes the brain to make changes to the body. If you remember, the brain is like a computer in that it needs its feedback in a certain manner before it will respond; it has to be absolutely perfect. The Vibrate-A-Way™ System utilizes the pattern of feedback into the body so that the brain then will respond to it. *Any deviation from this* will yield either no result at all or mediocre results at best. For those of you that want to be innovative and want to do it "your own way"—I see you. I know you because I am you! But, understand that this method will not work in the Vibrate-A-Way™ System. Therefore, either you are all in or please just save your time because it won't work. The technique you are about to learn to perform must stay pure and clean to be effective.

When you apply vibration, the tool you choose really doesn't matter. Don't spend $3,000 to buy a high-tech vibrational device when a $40 or $50 one will work. Any type of vibration works. If the device is slower and doesn't vibrate at a higher frequency, that's ok. It just might take a little bit longer in the application. Believe me, I know—I have tested many. The one factor that you do need to be aware of is that **vibration and percussion are two different things**. Most vibrational devices will have some percussion, but all the rage right now are the percussive massagers—you see athletes using them on their muscles on the sidelines, you see the television commercials, the Facebook ads. Those will not work as well as the vibration. So, you want to look at a device that has more vibration than it does percussion. It may be hard to find a device that is just basic vibration anymore.

When we apply vibration, there are a couple dos and don'ts. One, **you do not want to run the vibration over a bone**. The simplest reason is that it hurts. When vibration is applied, you need to make sure that your hands are feeling and protecting the bony landmarks near the application area. As we go through the protocols, I will be pointing this out to you. Next is pressure: how much pressure do you need, or how heavily do you push in on the device when you apply it to the body? The phrase that I use is "firm, not heavy." Let me try to clarify more. You should keep it at a pressure that if the person moved the area that you are working on, then your vibrational unit would also move with them; however, you don't want to grind the device into their body. Think of handshakes. We have all shaken somebody's hand: have you been a victim of a person who wanted to impress you with their firm grip, so they about broke your hand in two? Well, we don't want that kind of pressure, but there is a difference between a limp handshake and a firm handshake. Finally, a good rule of thumb is to listen to the recipient: they will tell you if the pressure is too hard or if it's good and adequate. Whenever you work on someone with Vibrate-A-Way™, communication is key.

Good phrases are: "that's too hard," "that's too soft" or, "you can press harder." So, always make sure that you are talking.

When we apply the vibration, we are going to make slow, steady passes along each muscle site. If you want to, you can use the "Mississippi" way of counting. I don't mean that people in Mississippi have different ways of counting; I mean, "One Mississippi, two Mississippi, three Mississippi..."—whatever you need to do to make sure that you have a nice, methodical pass of the vibrational device over the muscle. You can go by feeling of time or you can do a slow count, but what you don't want to do is to fly by it. You never want to pass over it really quickly. ***The general rule is to make a 3-second pass and repeat it 4 times***. So, keep this in your mind: 1) Four slow, steady passes 2) Be careful of bone 3) Firm but not heavy or forceful.

We will apply the technique bilaterally, which means to both sides; but pay attention to how many steps are performed on one side before repeating on the other side, as it varies. When we apply the protocols of Vibrate-A-Way™, there is a specific order that we use (there are several specific orders that we use!): We always start at the upper and then move to lower, followed by the post-protocol. Typically, with practice, the total application of a Vibrate-A-Way™ procedure should take you anywhere from 15 to 20 minutes.

Chapter 12:
Upper Body Protocols

Closely and accurately follow the diagrams and directions. This has all been laid out as clearly and concisely as a paint-by-number art project; so, you'll literally find numbers to follow with the specific sequential orders of all the protocols, as well as arrows demonstrating your vectors of vibration application. **It matters very much the direction in which you move that device!** That is part of the specificity of the brain. Lastly, you'll also notice circular symbols on some diagrams to indicate holding the vibration in that spot, as opposed to moving the device in a direction.

The numbers, diagrams and pictures are designed to be a quick reference, so you don't have to constantly look back into this text to perform the technique all the way through. Once you've read through all of these instructions, you can more confidently and simply use the photos/diagrams to help you follow the correct sequence until you've practiced it enough to have learned it. That may seem like a lot, now, but it won't take you long if you're performing it at least most days! To make it even simpler, we have wall charts available on our website, too.

Now that we've established some important ground rules for applying our vibration, let's begin by utilizing Vibrate-A-Way™ on the upper body. For this portion of application, the recipient should be seated on a treatment table, sideways chair or bench—

something that is stable but will allow access to their upper body, both front and back.

Standing behind your seated recipient, you are going to perform:

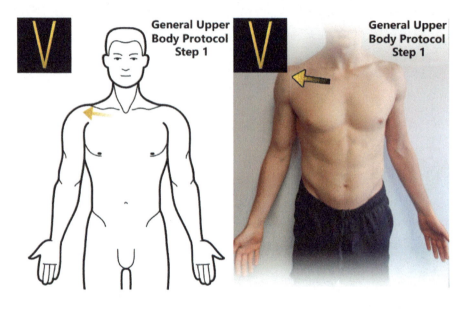

Step 1, the "pec" muscle. Feel and secure where the pec muscle is. Keep in mind, we also have ribs attached in this area, so you do not want to grind in. You want to make sure that you are cognizant of the sensitive rib area. Again, feedback from the recipient is important. You will take this vector on the "pec" muscle from the sternum, up diagonally toward the shoulder, making sure to go underneath the collarbone. It may help you to place your fingers lightly on the collarbone as you make your passes, to provide a bumper for the device. Also, do not apply the vibration onto the ball-and-socket joint of the shoulder, itself. You will want to stop as it gets close to that attachment of the muscle to the shoulder.

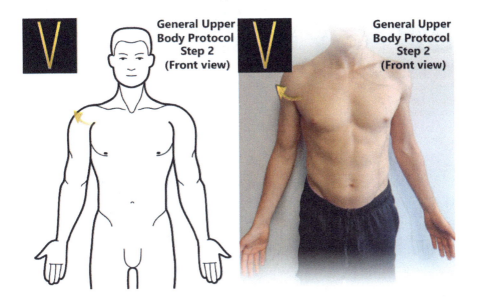

Step 2: You will be going around the side of the shoulder on the upper arm. These are the deltoid muscles. There are 3 branches of the deltoid muscle: the anterior, middle and posterior. Start at the front part where we associate the biceps being and go around the badge, like a badge of the shoulder. If you ever see those fancy military outfits where they have the shoulder badges or fringes hanging off in dress uniforms, that's what you are trying to go around. You want to make sure that you are beneath where the ball-and-socket is on the shoulder—just slightly below that. You will go from the front near the bicep area and take it around to the back where we have that upside-down "V" of where your armpit is.

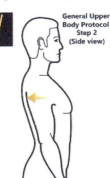

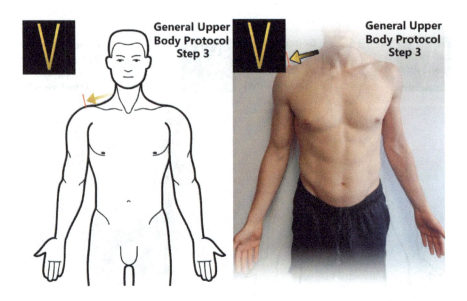

Step 3 is the upper trapezius. This is at the nape of the neck, down towards the shoulder. You'll be applying vibration to the upper "trap" and the SCM muscle. Be careful because, if you run your fingers down the length of that muscle, you will feel that you reach the bone of the shoulder pretty quickly. You are going to start from the base of the neck and only go about halfway out on the muscle. You don't want to go very long or you are going to hit the bone of the shoulder. It can help to lightly place your hand over the shoulder joint, to guard it from contact with the device. With this muscle, you can apply a little bit more pressure than maybe other areas because it is often very tight and is also a very thick muscle. Again, be sure to do the slow counts and be very deliberate. Sometimes, this area of the body is so small on some people/bodies that you don't really have a lot of room to move it on a line. What you will have to do in this case is place and hold it for the total time you would have done the passes.

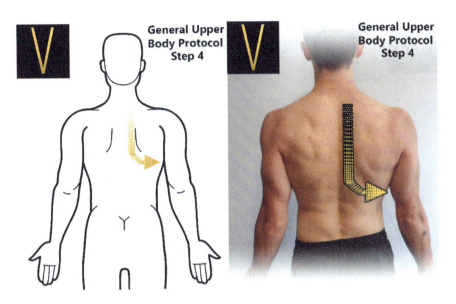

Step 4 will be around the shoulder blade. This can be a tricky one to find for some people because you have to go around the inner margin of the shoulder blade. This will apply vibration to various muscles like your rhomboids, your lower "trap," and different shoulder retractor muscles. You can make the shoulder blade more visible by asking the recipient to put their hand behind their back: that will reveal the margin of the shoulder blade. I will hook my fingers kind of around it and then have them put their arm back to where it should be. Then, I move my fingers off of that mark just a little bit, and I know that is where I am going to run the vibrational unit. You will kind of make a rough "J" or rounded "L" around that shoulder blade. Make sure you follow it all the way down and out. It's going to also be on the rib area, so when you get towards the bottom and outside of that shoulder blade, you need to be aware that you are on ribs, so you do not want to push too heavily.

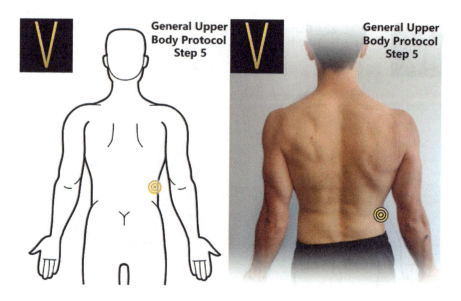

Step 5: You are going to target a specific spot of the waist: this is addressing the latissimus dorsi muscle. The latissimus dorsi is the largest muscle in the human body. It is located in the low back—or at least the belly of it is—and it comes up and attaches to the bottom of the shoulder blade. It actually attaches to the back of the humerus, where we would normally associate just the triceps being. This muscle is the prime mover of pulling your arm backwards. A lot of times when people rake leaves, they think their low back is what's hurting, but it's actually the shoulder muscle because that motion of raking is utilizing the latissimus dorsi. With the leaves being on grass, we deal with friction, and that creates extra work which wears out that muscle. So, there is just a little tidbit to know. Now, where you find this spot is just below the ribs and above the pelvic crest. You will feel a muscle that's really tight—you associate it with the low back—and you go off to the side until you don't feel it as much. Well, you want to be right in that margin where the muscle stops and it kind of goes

out to just the skin. You will place the device head there. This is one of the few where we don't do a motion but we leave it there. I generally leave it, because it is such a big muscle, for about 15 seconds.

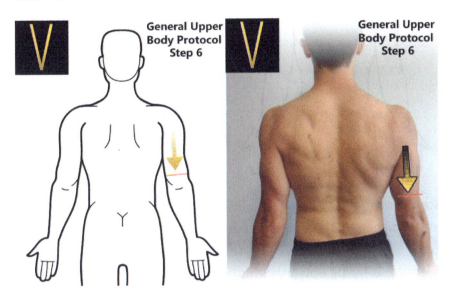

Step 6 has you going to the back of the humerus, or the back of the upper arm—the triceps. Your vector will be from where the upside-down "V" is—where the arm kind of meets the torso on the back of the arm, down, in a slow and deliberate manner. Always make sure that you don't hit the elbow. You may want to place your fingers over the elbow as a bumper against the device. That's a tender spot. Run the vibrational device until you hit, or come close to hitting, your fingers, and stop.

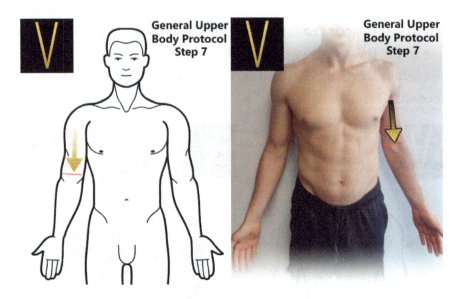

Step 7 takes you to the front of the upper arm, applying vibration to the bicep and the brachial radialus muscles. We all pretty much know where the bicep is. Ask the recipient to turn their hand so the palm is facing upwards: this helps to rotate out the humerus so that you can have more access to that bicep muscle. The motion will be downward as illustrated.

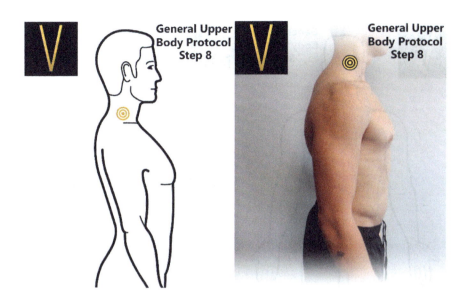

Step 8 is a spot at the side of the neck. Now, this one is tricky, so we are going to talk our way through this a little bit. You are going trace a line from where the collarbone meets the shoulder straight up the neck, so it's just slightly forward of the upper trapezius muscle. Make sure you are closer to the upper "trap" than you are to the throat area. This is important because you have carotid arteries and jugular veins. You do not want to be in the anterior portion of that. If in doubt, go more towards the back of the neck on the side. This is another "place and leave" application: hold for about 15 seconds. Pressure here should be more on the moderate side than the overly firm. It will create soreness if you leave it there for very long.

Repeat Steps 1-8 on the right side and then on the left side before proceeding to Step 9.

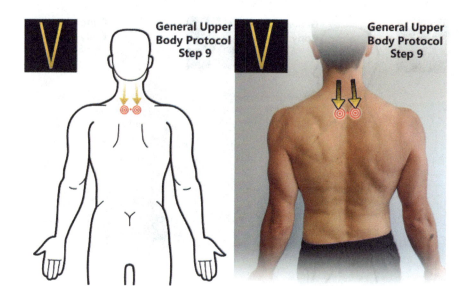

Lastly, **Step 9**. Stand behind the recipient and ask them to tuck in their chin so that it touches their chest. Run the vibrational unit, as pictured, on one side of the spine from just below the base of the skull where it connects to the neck, down to where the head connects to the shoulder. You're going to do that 3 to 4 times, slowly and deliberately, on both sides. If this makes the person feel dizzy, stop right away. They should not feel dizzy or experience vertigo. If that vertigo feeling does happen, find that little bump at the location of the spine where the mid-back meets the neck. Go to where that bump is and move out about an inch to either side: place the vibration there for 15 seconds. That's if they can't tolerate the vibration applied from the base of the skull, down.

Congratulations! You have performed the first protocol of the Vibrate-A-Way™ technique. What does this do? We expect the following improvements: 1) the head gets pulled back toward the midline, 2) the shoulders roll back and feel more pulled back, and 3) when the person is standing, their whole upper girdle has returned to the midline. Motion-wise, what we would like to see is more rotation in the neck, being able to turn the head left and right with less stiffness, less tightness. When muscles do abnormal work, people will describe that as tightness or stiffness. So, we should be able to see an increase in range of motion but *proper* motion—the right muscles doing the right jobs. In checking the shoulders, the recipient will ideally pass the collarbone test performed on each side after the upper protocol is complete (refer to Chapter 10). The arms should move freer and feel lighter.

This System takes time. The results that you are going to be looking for might be dramatic right away, and they might not. Remember: it's a process, not an event. So, look for those areas of improvement and realize that we must keep applying these procedures for the next 60 days.

Chapter 13:

Lower Body Protocols

We have just completed the upper body protocols; let's move now to the lower body. With this application, the recipient must first be lying on their back and then later on their stomach. Make sure the person is comfortable, but you also have to be cognizant that the surface they're lying on is not too soft. If they're lying on a very soft mattress, and you can see them sinking in whenever you apply pressure that might not be firm enough. So, it has to be comfortable yet firm enough not to alter their posture as you are applying the vibration. *Just as with the Upper Body Protocols, make 4 sweeps for each step for a slow count of 3 each sweep.*

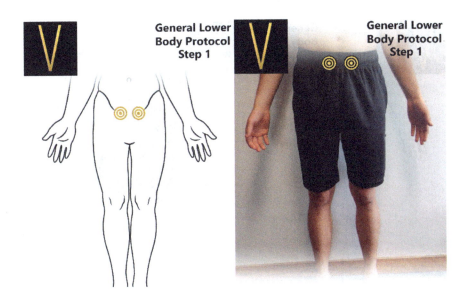

Step 1 will be both of the hip flexors, as shown. With the recipient lying on their back, you will feel for their pelvis. We call those pointy-outs, "hip bones," but that's actually a misnomer—that's the pelvic crest. On the side you're beginning with, you will locate a spot about an inch-and-a-half toward the midline from the pelvic crest/"hip bone" on that side, and that spot is the hip flexor. The hip flexors are another "place and leave" application; they are some of the strongest muscles of the human body, outside of the jaw, so this one I tend to hold the vibrational unit on each side for about 20 to 25 seconds. Apply on both sides.

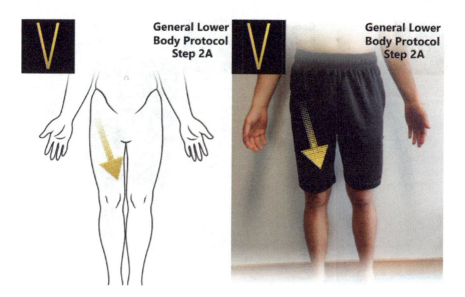

General Lower Body Protocol Step 2A

For Step 2, there is one application area but two different sweeps you'll be making with your device. After Step 1 is completed with the hip flexors, you'll move to the fronts of each leg—the "quads." The "quads" are short for quadriceps because there are 4 basic major muscle groups in the front of the leg. You will perform Step 2a and 2b on one leg and then the other, before progressing to Step 3. Whenever vibration is applied to the quads, the sensation will tend to be what I call a "tickle-tender-pressure-hurt." What I mean by that is—well, it's ticklish, it's kind of tender, it's just hard to describe. Some people will be very ticklish. It runs more toward being ticklish than it does hurting.

- **Step 2a**: Locate the very top of the quad on the outside, and you are going to make your vector like a diagonal that goes across the upper leg toward the inside of the knee. This will be most likely be ticklish: if the person is too sensitive to allow you to fluidly make the sweep across, then you can do a "place and leave" technique where you apply and hold the vibrational unit along the path, instead of one continuous pass. If even that is ticklish, one of the tricks I do is take my hand and go lower down on the quad and just kind of squeeze it a little--not a hard squeeze to make the person jump, but just a firm squeeze to add pressure. That pressure helps to diminish the tickling.

- **Step 2b**: At the top of the quad, your vector will be straight down toward the knee, as shown. Be sure to avoid the knee, using your hand as a bumper if necessary.

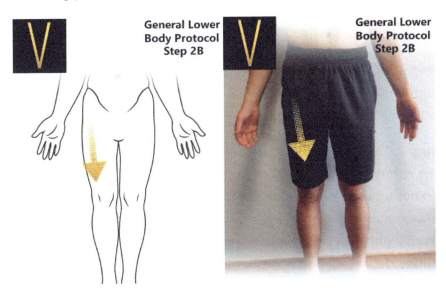

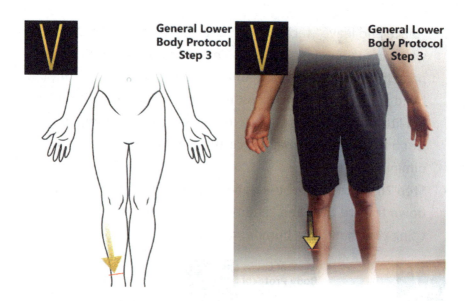

Step 3 & 4: You'll apply vibration to the anterior compartment and then the inside of the calf on one leg, and then again on the other leg before progressing.

Step 3: To the outside of each shin, you'll find muscle, and that is the anterior compartment of the leg. Feel along the entire shin: do not touch the bone with the device—that really hurts. So, I always put my finger on the shin and work it down as a bumper as I apply vibration on the muscle, from the top down toward the ankle. The anterior compartment is generally so tight that most people don't realize it. The vibration application feels like a pressure—almost like the sensation of a sausage exploding out of its casing when it's cooked. So, you always want to be cognizant of how the recipient is feeling.

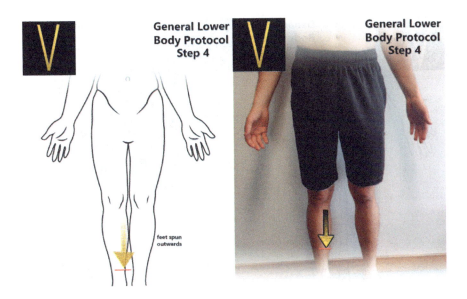

Step 4: Ask the recipient to spin their foot outward, so you can make a sweep with your device down the inside of the calf. Remember, on the shin part, it is bone, so you don't want to touch that with your device. You want to apply it on the inside where the muscle is, almost toward the back, to be safe. This sweep will be tender on most people. We only think of the calf as being on the back of the lower leg, but this inside part really gets tender.

That concludes the anterior, or front, part of the lower body. To recap, you should have applied vibration to both hip flexors, then both upper legs and, finally, both lower legs. The recipient should now lie on their stomach, face-down.

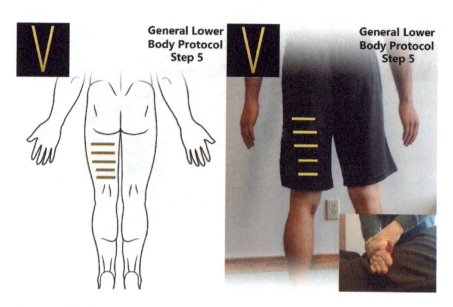

Step 5: The first thing that you want to address is the hamstrings. In my research and experimentation and finding the sequential order of all this, the hamstrings were the most difficult to decipher. You see, vibration on the hamstring muscle feels good, but it actually gave me no change in postural action. The muscle was still lengthened and tightened. It wasn't until I applied *stretch*: if you remember, proprioceptive nerves fire off with stretch as well as vibration. Therefore, what you will do is actually *stretch* the hamstring, but you will do this with your hand. Use the pinky side of your hand and angle your hand so it's like a knife edge. You know the old karate chop where you use that side of your hand? Well, it's not going to be straight up and down: it's going to be about a 45-degree angle. If you are right handed, you'll put your left hand on top to support your wrist. Make deliberate but short, quick thrusts at that 45-degree angle, about 3 or 4 times down the length of the hamstring, and you'll repeat those thrusts down the hamstring for a total of 2 to 3 times. You

don't want to go super deep: firm but not hard. We aren't trying to manipulate a bone. The purpose is to give a quick stretch reflex into the hamstring. Based on that, the brain will immediately relax that hamstring. Let the person's communication tell you. It is always better to start off light and then go firmer. Perform on hamstring of both legs.

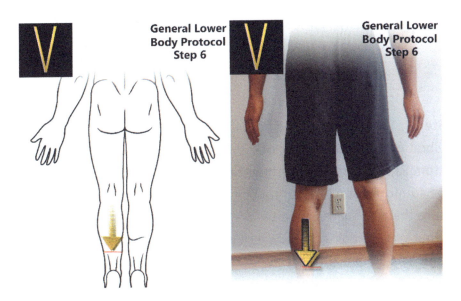

Step 6: Now, we're moving down the back of the legs to the calf muscles, just slightly off center to the outside. Your vector will go pretty straight from the top of the muscle, down. Be sure to pull off *before* you get to the Achilles tendon: you do not want to apply vibration on the Achilles tendon. Let me repeat: **DO NOT PUT VIBRATION ON THE ACHILLES TENDON.** You want to stop at least an inch to 2 inches before you get to it. Better to end short than to get on the tendon. Make a slow, steady path 3 to 4 times on calf of both legs.

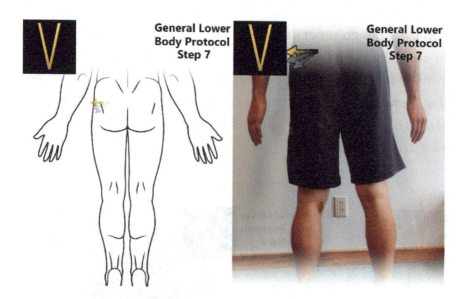

Step 7: The muscles of the pelvis: this will require applying the vibrational unit to the buttocks. With the recipient lying on their stomach, you first feel for their tailbone. Of course, they have to be comfortable with your touching them in this location. Make sure that you talk about it before you do it, and they know exactly what you are doing. Whenever I work on any patient, every single time I ask, "I am about ready to touch your buttocks to work on you. Do I have your permission?" It's always safe. Not just for legality but especially for courtesy and respect. Once you have the recipient's permission, feel for the tailbone and move your fingers out until you start to feel the muscles of the buttocks. From there, you are going to apply the vibration outward towards where the ball-and-socket is. There is a muscle there called the piriformis: it attaches from your tailbone and goes out to your ball-and-socket joint. This muscle is what rotates the legs outward; so, when your foot turns out, that's the muscle that's rotating the femur. The sciatic nerve sits underneath this muscle. When a person comes

into my clinic and talks about having a condition of the sciatic nerve, almost every time this muscle is too tight. When this muscle is tight, it compresses that nerve; so, we want to work on that. With this muscle, I do more than just 3 to 4 passes: I do 6 to 7. It is a big, powerful muscle, and you can apply a little more pressure here than most. Again, the comfort level of the recipient will determine that. Apply to both buttocks.

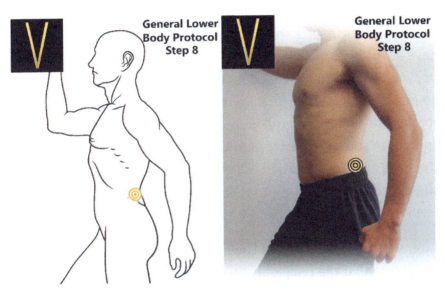

Step 8: Ask the recipient to lie on their side. It doesn't matter which side because you are going to do both. Do you remember when the recipient was seated, and you found that spot between the pelvis and the ribs? Well, you are going to find that spot again with the person lying on their side. Frankly, I don't know why the brain wants it this way, but it does. It needs to have that spot addressed while the person is seated and then at the very end of this protocol, it needs it again—but this time on the side. (As I've said before, it took me years of experimentation to basically

figure out the code of the brain for affecting/correcting posture. I do not know why, but that is part of the program of the brain.) It's very easy to find the muscle—just find that soft spot in between the pelvis and the ribs. Push down with your fingers, and you will feel the muscle, even through any kind of fat tissue or skin. Place the vibrational device there for about 15 seconds. There are people who have a very narrow gap between the pelvis and the ribs: in this case, make sure that you are on neither bone. You can try to angle the device so the contact point is smaller. Maybe you have a smaller attachment head on your vibrational device; if you do, you can use that. If that does not do it, then you will want to go just slightly anterior (toward the front) of that spot because that gap becomes bigger. If you can't safely wedge it in onto the spot, then you go more forward toward the stomach until you get that nice gap. The vibration will travel; it will not be as intense and site-specific, but it will get to that muscle to release the pelvis even more.

After you are done with the Lower Protocols, it is important to make sure that the recipient gets up, walks around a little and moves about to note any differences in how they feel; this also allows you to make observations about their posture and gait.

Chapter 14:
Post-Protocols

The goal of the Post Protocols is trifold: to level the pelvis, to increase shoulder motion, and to create a longer, freer stride while walking.

Step 1 consists of three individual steps in order to level the pelvis. Ask the recipient to lie on their side. Complete all three steps on one side; ask them to turn, and then complete all three steps on their other side.

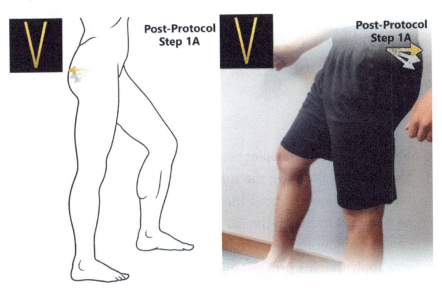

- **Step 1a**: Locate the ball-and-socket joint at the side of the hip with your fingers. Beginning at that point, you'll have three vectors: one straight from the ball-and-socket joint toward the tailbone/sacrum (do not apply vibration directly onto the tailbone); another at more of an angle toward the mid-tailbone; thirdly, about a 45-degree angle toward the bottom of the tailbone. This helps to ensure adequate coverage of the pelvic muscles. Perform three sets of that set of three vectors for the usual three seconds each path.

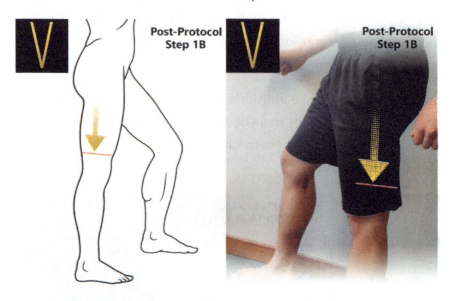

- **Step 1b**: With the recipient still lying on that same side, run the unit straight down the side of the thigh, from below the hip to a few inches above the side of the knee, for three passes. This muscle is the iliotibial band, or the "IT band," and can feel tender for the recipient, so be careful of the pressure you apply that it's firm but not hard.

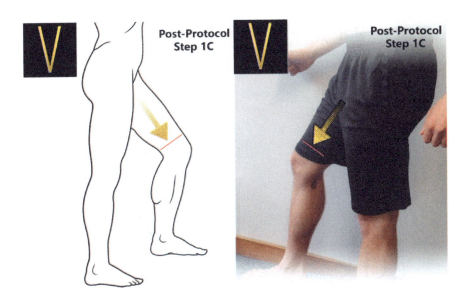

- **Step 1c**: The line of vibration you just applied to the outer thigh for that leg, you'll repeat for the *inner* thigh on the *other* leg. They can remain on their side for this; just ask them to move their leg back to give you clear access to their inner thigh. Alternatively, they can lie on their back, straighten one leg, and bend the other in like a frog-leg, but it's usually easier to stay lying on their side. Again, three passes straight down, ending above the knee. This is often another "tickle-pressure-tender-hurt" muscle, so sometimes the place-and-hold method is more comfortable for the recipient.

Step 2 consists of two individual steps to again address the latissimus dorsi muscle, along with the QL. The recipient will lie on one side for both steps, then ask them to lie on their other side to complete both steps again.

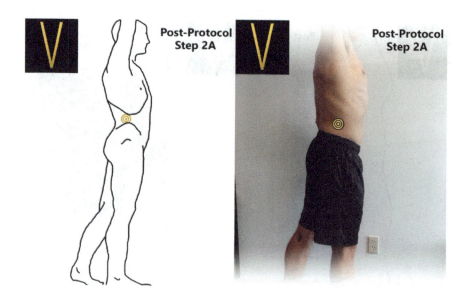

- **Step 2a**: For this step, you'll simply repeat Step 8 from the Lower Protocols. This application of vibration to this spot of the "lat" may seem redundant, but the brain is so particular and specific that performing this step then and again during this sequence is necessary for the results sought after. This step also applies vibration to the quadratus lumborum, or "QL."

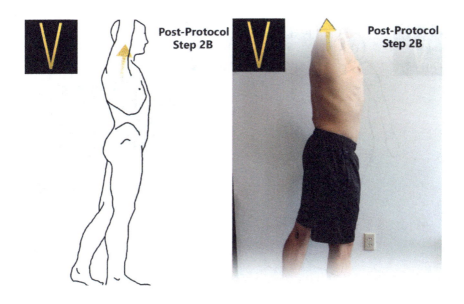

- **Step 2b**: Ask the recipient to bring their arm up in a comfortable position over their head. With their ribs more exposed, you can feel at the crest of the ribs, going up, the "lat" muscle. With your device, you'll follow that muscle and apply vibration from around the middle of the side the ribs, on up to just behind the armpit and the first quarter of the arm near the triceps. This section of the "lat" may be—again—very tender, so communicate with your recipient to adjust pressure; also, do not push too hard on the rib area. Make three passes on each side, as you've been doing.

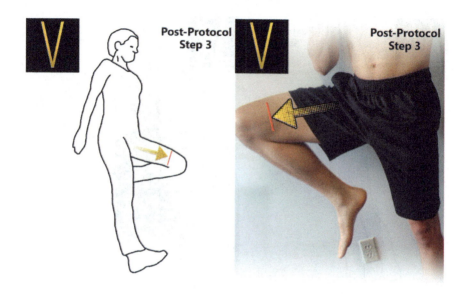

- **Step 3:** Ask your Vibrate-A-Way™ recipient to lie on their back and bend one leg out to frog-leg, again to give access to the inner thigh. You'll be repeating Step 1c on each inner thigh: apply the unit to the upper inner thigh, straight down to above the knee, three passes each leg. This step can help to smooth out and lengthen stride.

Once Step 3 is completed, ask the recipient to walk for you. Observe freedom of movement and smoothness of gait, if their stride is of more of a normal length. Maybe they're walking more softly or quietly?

Also observe their upper body: some people's brains will maintain a posture of being rolled forward or kind of "crumpled" in the middle, if you will. If this is the case for your recipient, complete optional step 4.

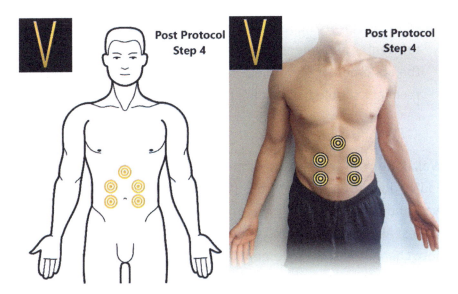

Step 4 is another sequence or a pattern of the brain. Why it sometimes wants it this way, I don't know. You'll perform this step in three parts on the abdomen: the top center, two points on one side, then two on the other. All steps are pictured together but performed sequentially. Notice the "house" pattern, as shown.

- **Step 4a**: This is the roof of the house. Go to where the xiphoid process, or the base of the sternum, is and you can feel that soft tissue muscle just below it. Place and hold the vibrational unit there for about 10 seconds, carefully avoiding the bone.
- **Step 4b**: Now you'll make the walls of the house, one side and then the other. Follow the margin of the rib to one side, moving down and out from the midline about 2 inches. Place the unit there, being careful not to place it on the rib, itself, and hold for 10 seconds. Then, go down vertically about another 2 inches, as pictured. Place and hold the vibration

there as before. Repeat on the other side. So, you have the top center placement, and you have 2 spots on each side on the abdomen. If "crumpled" or rolled forward, before, your recipient should be standing taller and straighter, now.

Well done! You've performed the Vibrate-A-Way™ technique! As you've done after each protocol, be sure to ask the recipient to walk and move around, being aware of how their body feels and moves. Also, you'll want to observe their gait and posture and note changes and improvements since before the application.

Analyze what you've noticed, before and after, and look for these same things before the next session.

Final Thoughts

Hopefully, by this point you have been able to utilize the Vibrate-A-Way™ protocols and have seen the changes in your loved ones (and yourself, if they've performed the technique on you, too!). It is important to understand that the Vibrate-A-Way™ Program is a 60-day program. The brain will give up control of its previous posture after about 60 calendar days.

What is common with this program is that the immediate results are so distinctly felt and seen that many people can't believe it—they cannot grasp just what has happened to them: the way they look, how much more freely and easily they can move, and the often dramatic relief from their pain. I've witnessed countless patients joyfully crying, calling their loved ones from my treatment room. The immediate results can be quite significant—especially if somebody has tried everything under the sun and has not had much success. But what happens is the first 70% of change is very noticeable; the last 30% isn't. That is why it is so imperative to continue with the 60-day program.

What I recommend for frequency during the program is, at least for the first one or two weeks, you do it every day. Keep in mind that it only takes 15 to 20 minutes of your day, especially with repetition and practice. You can do it at least once a day: you generally cannot perform the protocols too much. There is no downside to doing it twice a day or three times a day. What you have to realize is that, in the beginning, there will be a dramatic tug-of-war between the corrected posture/corrected movement and the brain's accommodated posture/accommodated motion. Remember, the brain wants you stable, and that is the most important thing in the world to the brain. So, it's not going to give up easily and just say, "Oh, I'm sorry. Sure, we will do it your way." No, the brain is more resilient than that, and things that are a blessing can also be a curse.

Even though the brain is resilient, and that helps us in so many avenues of healthcare with musculoskeletal posture and movement, sometimes that goes against us. You are going to feel good and then you are going to feel like you reverted back—it goes back and forth. Try to pay attention and notice the level of pain and discomfort. Is it not as intense? Does it not last as long? Maybe it's changed. I often talk to my patients about getting out of the pain mode. See, the reason why we originally see a practitioner is because we hurt. It hurts to move a certain way. It hurts to do a certain thing. Pain is the number one reason, but if you focus instead on *function*—and you can correct abnormal function—then most times the pain will leave. Remember, pain is not a disease; pain is a *symptom*. We know that we must kill off the virus of a common cold, and we know that the symptoms are coughing, sneezing, and runny nose. We may take medications to help with those symptoms, but we don't focus on getting rid of the symptoms only. It's about getting rid of the virus. It's about truly going back to the root cause of the symptom, and in our case, that symptom is pain. When the root cause is addressed and corrected, that pain resolves. Those who are caught inside the Pain Matrix are futilely stuck, focusing on and trying to address only the symptom of pain; but Vibrate-A-Way™ is the future's solution to musculoskeletal pain and dysfunction.

When you analyze your progress, track your posture with your pictures and observe your gait with your videos; but, most importantly, learn to become self-aware of how you're feeling and moving during your everyday activities. Are you noticing that it doesn't hurt so much to do your favorite hobby? Or perhaps when you are done with a day's work, you don't feel totally spent and wiped out and in pain? Take notice of those things. You and you alone are responsible for your quality of life. In healthcare, we have made great strides in longevity—extending a person's life; but if you take a look at everything around you, you know that healthcare has dropped the ball when it comes to *quality* of life. And that, my friends, is the secret of Vibrate-A-Way™. The Vibrate-A-Way™ program was designed to help improve your *quality* of life. After all, if you can move better and be in less pain, you can do more things. You can do those things that you love like walking long distances, playing a sport, going hunting, playing with the grandchildren, whatever it might be. You can do them for longer durations and in less pain. You have a better quality of life. So, pay attention to how you move and feel while doing everyday activities and the things that bring you joy.

Another thing to remember about Vibrate-A-Way™ is that the corrections are being made by the brain. As the brain is basically recalibrating itself, you need to do the program within the prism of your normal life—while doing what you have always done and what you want to do. As I have said previously, any fool can make you feel better by telling you to stay stationary and never actually do anything that might cause you pain; but for your brain to make these changes with the different synergies of movement and action, it has to do it in the correct posture. The only way it's going to know to do that is if we do those common, everyday things. Then we can correct the posture and movement as we go, within the prism of your normal life. Isn't that why you bought this book? The Pain Matrix had you focusing on the pain and dysfunction instead of function. If your shoulder hurts, quit trying to figure how the zebra got in the bathtub. We need to get it out. We need to improve the quality of your life, and if you follow this 60-day program—like countless others—my hope is that you will see those positive changes.

You see, the Vibrate-A-Way™ 60-day program is not a product. No! Vibrate-A-Way™ is a *movement*. Vibrate-A-Way™ is a cause. *Its name is the Pain-Free Initiative*. I'm not looking to sell a book. I'm looking to get people to join us in the Pain-Free Initiative: a cause where we don't accept the status quo of having to live in pain, of believing this is as good as it gets as we get older, or blaming an injury from 25 years ago and being given a prescription—all fragments of the Pain Matrix so many are trapped inside by way of thinking and doing. A lifetime of prescription drugs, surgeries, or endless chiropractic appointments will not eradicate the problem. This is why I want to promote and spread the new system of Vibrate-A-Way™ and the Pain-Free Initiative: to revolutionize and raise the bar on standard healthcare and bring awareness of the Pain Matrix to you and to everyone, offering an escape and a better life as a result.

I encourage you to go to our website www.vibrateaway.com. We offer videos and more information about the Pain-Free Initiative and how you can join and get involved. If you know somebody who hurts, who has been dealing with issues with their body for years and has tried "everything," tell them about us. In fact, tell three people and ask them to do the same once their lives have been changed. This is so very important! If each impacted life can impact three more lives, the Pain-Free Initiative will reach around the world, successfully improving the lives and spread of love everywhere!

If you've learned and practiced all I've shared in this book and would like to learn how you can make a difference in people's lives with the Vibrate-A-Way™ system, look for our Core Certification course, taking knowledge and application of our program to higher levels.

We're ever researching and synthesizing data, in order to further tap into the power of vibration and the brain and offer more solutions to pain and dysfunction. We have just scratched the surface of what the brain can do. It can do so much! It is harnessing this power that, I believe, can aid us on our quest to eradicate musculoskeletal problems and potentially many other health problems. And it is through the use of vibration and frequency that we can aid the brain in making our health better. Tesla said, "If you want to find the secrets of the universe, think in terms of energy, frequency and vibration." He was right: everything travels in waves, everything is about frequency and vibration. It is the ability to harness this power that can make revolutionary breakthroughs in our society. In my heart of hearts, I know that the application of vibration to the human body in this, the Vibrate-A-Way™ 60-day program, is one of those revolutionary breakthroughs.

May God bless you, may God protect you, and may God give you good health. After all, God is the Physician of Physicians; I am the guy to whom this was revealed. Thank you for reading with an open mind, and I hope we can continue on this journey together.

Made in the USA
Columbia, SC
20 September 2023

23105760R00065